Handbook on Cerebral Artery Dissection

Frontiers of Neurology and Neuroscience

Vol. 20

Series Editor

J. Bogousslavsky *Lausanne*

KARGER

Handbook on Cerebral Artery Dissection

Volume Editors

R.W. Baumgartner *Zürich*
J. Bogousslavsky *Lausanne*
V. Caso *Perugia*
M. Paciaroni *Perugia*

35 figures, 2 in color, and 24 tables, 2005

KARGER

Basel · Freiburg · Paris · London · New York ·
Bangalore · Bangkok · Singapore · Tokyo · Sydney

Prof. Dr. Ralf W. Baumgartner
Neurologische Klinik
Frauenklinikstrasse 26
CH–8091 Zürich (Switzerland)

Prof. Dr. Julien Bogousslavsky
Department of Neurology
CHUV
CH–1011 Lausanne (Switzerland)

Dr. Dr. Valeria Caso
Department of Neuroscience
University of Perugia
Via Enrico dal Pozzo
IT–06126 Perugia (Italy)

Dr. Maurizio Paciaroni
Stroke Unit, University of Perugia
Ospedale Silvestrini
Sant' Andrea delle Fratte
IT–06126 Perugia (Italy)

Library of Congress Cataloging-in-Publication Data

Handbook on cerebral artery dissection / volume editors, R.W. Baumgartner
... [et al.].
p. ; cm. – (Frontiers of neurology and neuroscience ; v. 20)
Includes bibliographical references and index.
ISBN 3-8055-7986-1 (hard cover : alk. paper)
1. Cerebral arteries–Dissection–Handbooks, manuals, etc. I.
Baumgartner, R. W. (Ralf W.) II. Series.
[DNLM: 1. Vertebral Artery Dissection. 2. Cerebral
Arteries–physiopathology. 3. Cervical Vertebrae–blood supply. WL 355 H2366 2005]
RD594.2.H36 2005
617.4′71–dc22

2005021723

Bibliographic Indices. This publication is listed in bibliographic services.

www.karger.com
Printed in Switzerland on acid-free paper by Reinhardt Druck, Basel
ISSN 1660–4431
ISBN 3–8055–7986–1

Contents

Preface

This volume of *Frontiers of Neurology and Neuroscience* is devoted to cerebral artery dissection, a field in which much progress has been made in the last decade. Thus, the idea of this book was to bring together experts from all over the world to give an overview about the present knowledge and future research directions of this still poorly understood disease.

In the first chapter an animal model of carotid dissection is elaborated. In the next six chapters, epidemiology and the current knowledge and hypotheses about possible mechanisms of spontaneous and traumatic cervical artery dissection are presented. In particular, the association of cervical artery dissection with connective tissue abnormalities in skin and arteries, genetic approaches and vasodilation are discussed. The next two chapters describe the clinical manifestations of cervical internal carotid and vertebral artery dissection. The possibilities and limitations of the main diagnostic tools, ultrasound, CT, MR imaging and angiography, are the subject of chapters 10–12. An overview about the prognosis, thrombolytic and antithrombotic therapy of cervical artery dissection is given in chapters 13–15. Intracranial cerebral artery dissection is discussed in the last chapter.

It is our hope that this volume will contribute to efforts linking clinical and basic science, provide the reader with new insights and perspectives and stimulate his interest in this fascinating vascular disease.

The editors thank the authors who have made this volume possible.

Ralf W. Baumgartner
Julien Bogousslavsky
Valeria Caso
Maurizio Paciaroni

Baumgartner RW, Bogousslavsky J, Caso V, Paciaroni M (eds): Handbook on Cerebral Artery Dissection. Front Neurol Neurosci. Basel, Karger, 2005, vol 20, pp 1–11

Animal Models of Cervical Artery Dissection

Takeshi Okamoto, Shigeru Miyachi, Jun Yoshida

Department of Neurosurgery, Nagoya University Graduate School of Medicine, Nagoya, Japan

Abstract

We developed a canine model of arterial dissection and serially observed morphological changes angiographically and histopathologically to clarify the causes and mechanisms resulting in dissecting aneurysm formation or arterial occlusion. Intimal defects of various sizes and shapes were made on the arterial walls to provide an entry zone for dissection, so as to simulate the extent of arterial wall injury. Our experimental model showed angiographic and histopathological changes similar to those in clinical cases. As for our initial findings immediately after lesioning, either a double shadow (pseudolumen) or stenosis of the affected artery, due to compression from the subadventitial hematoma, was observed in the angiograms of all lesions. In some lesions with a pseudolumen, a dissecting aneurysm developed subsequently. Some arteries showing focal occlusion recanalized, and stenosis spontaneously improved. Very small dissections resulted in spontaneous healing, while a large intimal entry zone caused stenotic lesions. However, a medium-sized entry zone (4–6 mm) may induce aneurysm formation. The different features of dissection may be caused by the characteristics of flow into the subadventitial cavity and by thrombogenesis. Morphological changes after arterial dissection were closely related to the extent of intimal injury, suggesting that the size of the intimal entry zone may determine whether or not a dissecting aneurysm is formed.

Extracranial carotid artery dissection most often is related to penetrating or blunt trauma to the neck, or to intraoral trauma [1–3]. Hyperextension and rotation of the head may stretch the carotid artery against an upper cervical vertebra or a prominent styloid process, while in other situations abrupt severe neck flexion may directly compress the internal carotid artery between the angle of the mandible and the upper cervical spine [3, 4]. Similarly, hyperrotation of the neck can induce vertebral artery dissection at the craniocervical junction [5–7]. Such excessive motion of the neck causes shearing stress against the inner layers of vascular wall resulting in an intimal tear or mural contusion; then blood can enter the media at the site of intimal injury and dissect the arterial wall [8–11]. Nontraumatic causes of dissection include fibromuscular dysplasia, Marfan syndrome, syphilis, hypertension, and arteriosclerosis [10, 12].

Arterial dissection can follow either or both of two clinical patterns: dissecting aneurysm presenting with hemorrhage, or stenosis or occlusion with ischemic symptoms [13]. However, the factors that define morphological and clinical characteristics of dissection are unsettled. We therefore developed a canine model of arterial dissection and serially observed morphological changes angiographically and histopathologically to clarify the causes and mechanisms resulting in dissecting aneurysm formation or arterial occlusion [14].

Experimental Models of Arterial Dissection

Dissection can occur in any artery throughout the body. Many points of uncertainty or controversy remain with respect to etiology, pathogenesis, and treatment strategy. To answer some of these questions, particularly for aortic dissection, various experimental models have been used. Wilens et al. [15] ligated several feeding branches to the aorta in mongrel dogs, while Takeoka [16] infiltrated mitomycin C into the media of the canine aorta, but in both studies, only medial edematous change developed, not spontaneous dissection. Dogs with renal hypertension also failed to develop aortic dissection [16]. Takeoka [16] created a traumatic dissection model by surgical methods and succeeded in producing an aortic lesion with a pseudolumen, but surgical lesioning has not been used to produce carotid dissection until now. To our knowledge, ours is the first report of an experimental model of carotid artery dissection.

Experimental Model of Carotid Artery Dissection

Our experimental dissection model [14] showed angiographic and histopathological changes similar to those in clinical cases [1, 3, 4, 8, 10, 11, 17, 18]. As for initial findings after producing dissection by intimal injury, either a double shadow (pseudolumen) or stenosis of the affected artery, due to compression from the subadventitial hematoma, was observed in angiograms of all lesions. In some lesions with a pseudolumen, a dissecting aneurysm developed subsequently. Some arteries showing focal occlusion recanalized, and stenosis spontaneously improved. Details of our experimental model is as follows.

Materials and Methods

In our experimental model [14], artificial dissection with intimal injury was induced physically on the common carotid artery of mongrel dogs (body weight, 16–20 kg), with the intent to mimic traumatic dissection. This experiment was performed using a protocol approved by the Nagoya University Animal Care Committee. The animals were anesthetized with an intramuscular injection of ketamine hydrochloride (3 mg/kg) and an intravenous injection of pentobarbital (5 mg/kg), and then intubated and allowed to breathe room air spontaneously. General anesthesia was maintained with additional doses of pentobarbital, as required. Each surgical procedure was performed under sterile conditions with the aid of an operating microscope.

In common carotid arteries, a small incision limited to the adventitial layer was made following the placement of vascular clamps distally and proximally. The adventitia was then dissected from the media using a thin probe passed through the adventitial incision. After sufficient dissection between the two layers, varying longitudinally oriented intimal defects were incised in the intima, including the media. These steps were meticulously performed using small scissors inserted through the adventitial window. The intimal defect was created at a point some distance distal to the adventitial incision to ensure intact adventitia, where blood entered the dissected cavity. The adventitial incision was then tightly closed, and the vascular clamps were removed (fig. 1).

As an intimal entry zone simulates the extent of arterial wall injury, intimal defects of various sizes and shapes were made on the arterial walls. In 47 cases, elliptical intimal defects were made, extending longitudinally between 2 and 8 mm [subgroup I-A (2 mm), I-B (4 mm), I-C (6 mm), and I-D (8 mm)]. In 17 cases, the intimas were cut longitudinally for a length between 4 and 8 mm [subgroups II-A (4 mm), II-B (6 mm), and II-C (8 mm)]. The width of the ellipse was equal to half of the arterial diameter (approximately 2 mm) in all lesions of this shape. The incised lengths were exactly measured and confirmed by a scale. In total, 64 experimental dissections were created on the arterial walls of 34 mongrel dogs (table 1).

Immediately after completion of these procedures, external changes in the dissected portion were observed macroscopically. A carotid angiogram was then performed by the Seldinger method. In all cases, a second angiogram followed 30 min to 2 h later to determine the acute changes, including any improvement in the stenosis, progressive occlusion, and recanalization. Follow-up angiography was performed after 1 week and 3 months. No anticoagulation or antiplatelet medication was administered before, during, or following creation of the dissections. After the final follow-up angiogram or following an animal's death from complications, dissected arteries were harvested for histopathological examination by light microscopy and scanning electron microscopy.

Results

Morphological Changes (Table 1)

Immediately after recanalization all lesions showed abrupt formation of a dense subadventitial hematoma due to influx of blood through the intimal entry zone (fig. 2–4). These usually were massive and frequently extended not only distally but also proximally from the intimal entry zone along the plane of

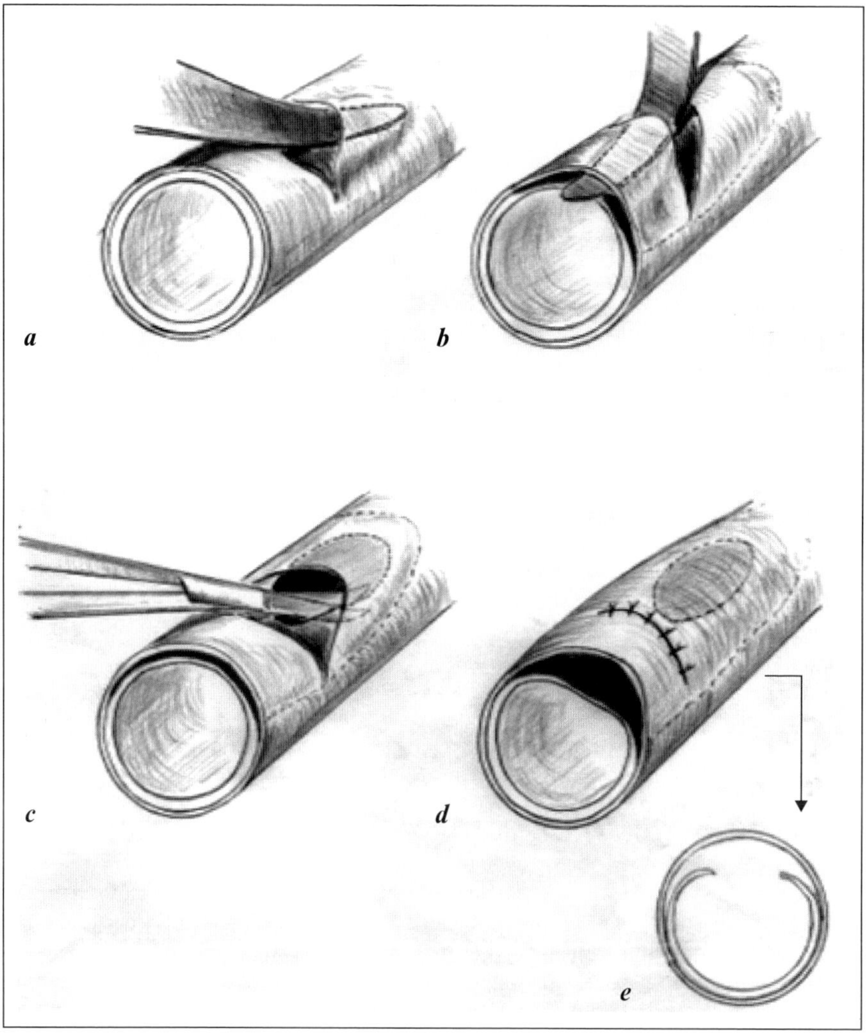

Fig. 1. The method used for creating experimental dissection. In canine common carotid arteries, a small incision limited to the adventitial layer was made (***a***). Then the adventitia was dissected from the media using a thin probe passed through the adventitial incision (***a, b***). After sufficient dissection between the two layers, a longitudinal slit-like or elliptical defect was cut in the intima (***c***). Then the adventitial incision was tightly closed (***d***). (***e***) Cross-section corresponding to (***d***).

Table 1. Summary of angiographic changes (acute/subacute/chronic stage)

Size of incision	Normal	Aneurysm	Aneurysm + stenosis	Stenosis	Occlusion	Failed to follow-up	Total
I-A	0/11/13	0/1/0	0/0/0	14/2/0	0/0/0	0/0/1	14
I-B	0/3/7	0/8/6	0/1/0	12/1/0	1/0/0	0/0/0	13
I-C	0/0/2	0/0/0	3/6/2	5/4/4	2/0/0	0/0/2	10
I-D	0/0/0	0/0/0	3/0/0	5/0/0	2/10/10	0/0/0	10
II-A	0/5/6	0/2/1	0/0/0	7/0/0	0/0/0	0/0/0	7
II-B	0/3/3	0/1/1	0/1/0	5/0/0	0/0/0	0/0/1	5
II-C	0/0/2	0/1/0	0/3/2	3/1/1	2/0/0	0/0/0	5

adventitial separation. The initial angiogram demonstrated stenotic change in the artery in all lesions, including total occlusion (fig. 4). The stenotic change was particularly marked at the site of the intimal entry zone, and in about 60% lesions a subadventitial pseudolumen was visualized, showing influx of contrast medium (fig. 2, 3). On comparing groups according to characteristics of the intimal entry zone, severe stenotic changes most often were found in groups I-C and I-D. Groups with longitudinal incisions showed less extensive subadventitial hematoma formation than groups with elliptical incisions. The second angiogram in the acute stage was performed in all cases within 2 h following the initial one. No pseudolumen was opacified, and of the 7 lesions with total occlusion of the artery on the initial angiogram, 6 showed recanalization; in 49 of 57 lesions stenosis had improved slightly.

All animals underwent follow-up angiography at 1 week (subacute stage). Angiograms at this subacute stage demonstrated morphological changes that varied by size of intimal entry zone. In 79% with group I-A, stenosis had normalized and arterial contour was smooth. However, lesions with group I-B resulted in aneurysm formation in 62%. All lesions with group I-C showed persistent stenosis (fig. 3), and 60% were associated with aneurysm (fig. 2). All lesions with group I-D were associated with complete occlusion of the artery (fig. 4). As for groups with longitudinal incisions (II-A, II-B, and II-C) no significant relationship was found between incision length and morphological change (table 1). Aneurysms were berry shaped and limited to the area of the intimal entry zone (fig. 2).

Sixty lesions were followed for 3 months (chronic stage). One dog died because of systemic complications, and 3 died of repeated rupture of aneurysms within 2 weeks. Postmortem histopathological study showed that the rupture points were found at the top of the aneurysms, not the site of surgical access.

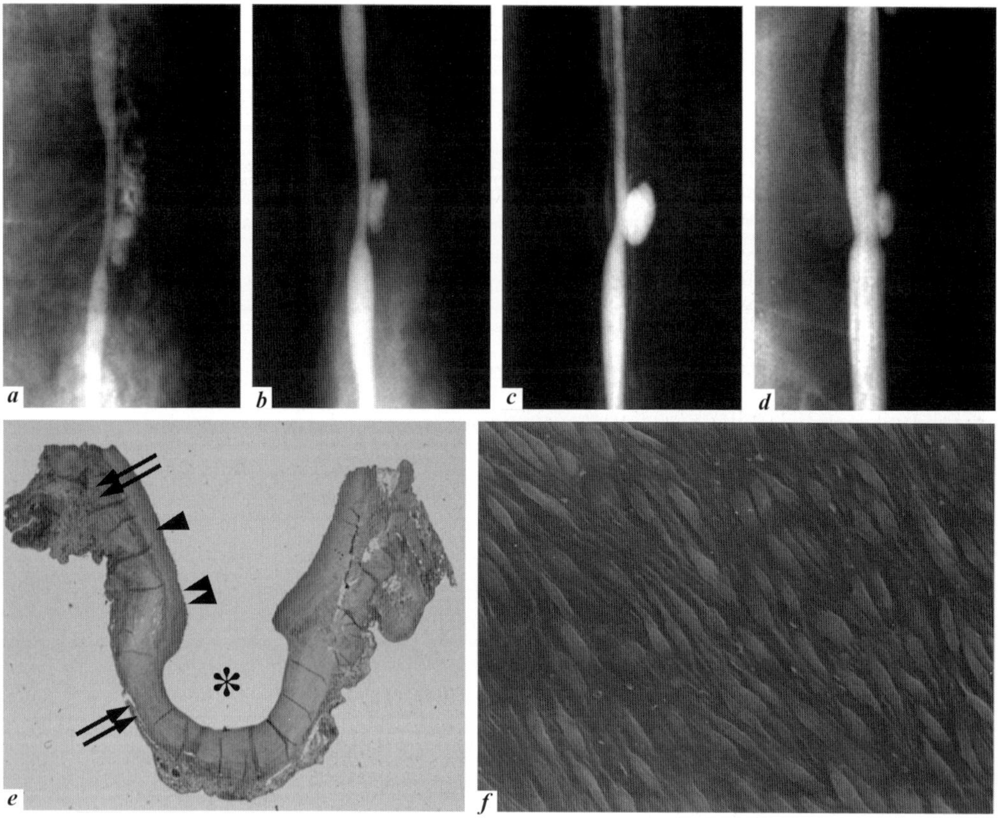

Fig. 2. An example of aneurysm formation. An angiogram shows a double shadow due to a massive adventitial hematoma immediately following lesioning (***a***), and a subadventitial hematoma had acquired the characteristics of an aneurysmal pouch 2 h later (***b***), becoming a saccular aneurysm 1 week later (***c***). The size of the aneurysm decreased in the chronic stage (3 months later) (***d***). Histopathological study demonstrated that the inner layer of the aneurysm dome (asterisk) was covered with organized clots and fully endothelialized in the chronic stage (***e***). Elastica van Gieson, original magnification ×5 (the adventitia, media, and intima are indicated by double arrows, arrowhead, and double arrowheads, respectively). (***f***) Scanning electron microscopy showed endothelialization (original magnification ×700).

These cases belonged to subgroup I-B, I-C, and II-C, respectively, and no relationship was seen between size of intimal defect, aneurysm size, and point of rupture. In lesions including aneurysms, the aneurysms were unchanged in size or slightly smaller (fig. 2); no aneurysm showed enlargement. Stenoses observed in the subacute stage had improved remarkably (fig. 3). No complete occlusion had recanalized.

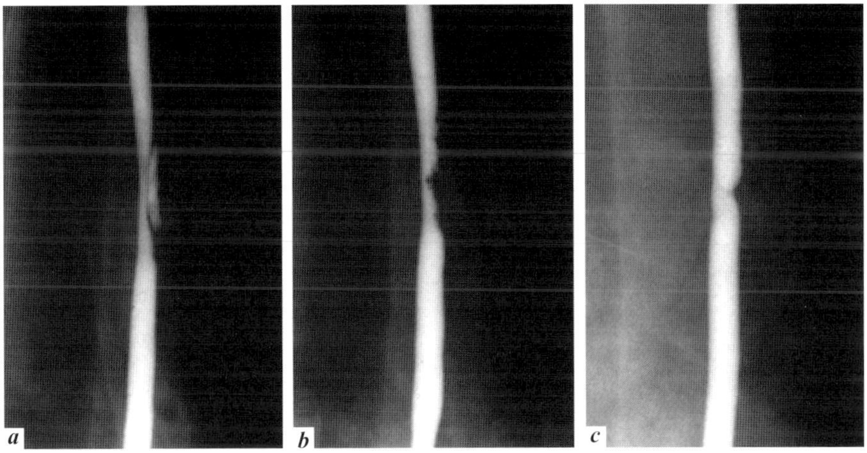

Fig. 3. An example of persistent stenosis. An angiogram demonstrated that a subadventitial hematoma compressed the arterial lumen just after lesioning (***a***). Two hours later the subadventitial hematoma had spontaneously thrombosed, but it still compressed the arterial lumen (***b***). In the chronic stage stenosis improved (***c***).

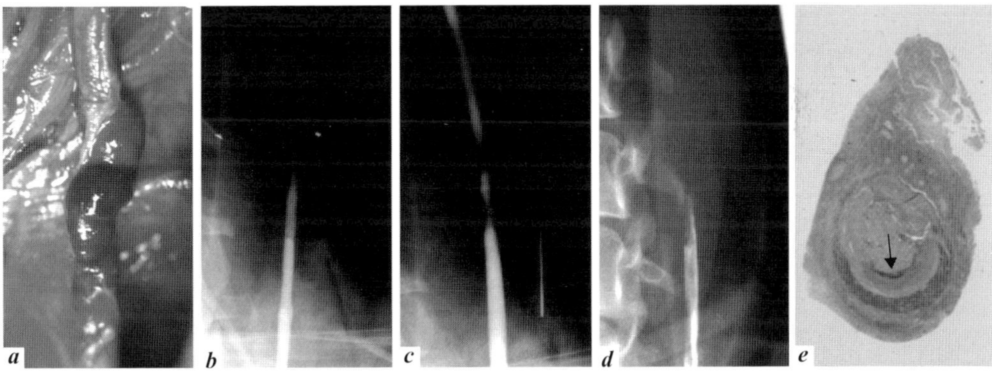

Fig. 4. An example of occlusion. Immediately after lesioning the arterial lumen was compressed and acquired a serpentine configuration with a subadventitial hematoma on macroscopic inspection (***a***) and occlusion in an angiogram (***b***). The vessel lumen transiently recanalized after 2 h (***c***), but occluded again in the subacute stage (***d***). (***e***) The subadventitial hematoma, which already was organized, compressed the arterial lumen to present a crescentic cross-sectional profile in a histological section (elastica van Gieson, original magnification ×5, arrow demonstrates the compressed arterial lumen).

Histopathological Changes

On transversely oriented cross-sections, the dissection cavity was evident microscopically as a crescent-shaped cleft between adventitia and media, filled with fresh clot in the acute stage. Serial sections indicated that clots extended both distal and proximal to the intimal entry zone. In lesions with persistent stenosis, subadventitial clots were partially organized in the chronic stage. In lesions with aneurysm formation, a portion of the intimal entry zone extended to the orifice of the aneurysm. In cases of aneurysm with stenosis, the external protrusion of the aneurysm was small and clots in the surrounding subadventitial space formed the lateral wall of the aneurysm (fig. 2). The inner layer of the aneurysm dome was covered with fresh thin clots in the acute stage and was fully endothelialized in the chronic stage; the latter was clearly demonstrated by scanning electron microscopy (fig. 2).

Statistical Analysis

Statistical analysis among groups defined by incision size and shape was performed using Fisher's exact probability test.

On comparison by size of intimal entry zone, the likelihood of aneurysm formation was significantly greater in the group I-B than I-A and I-D ($p < 0.01$). The lesions in the group I-D were more likely to occlude the artery than a shorter entry zone ($p < 0.01$). Longitudinal incisions showed no obvious morphological differences according to length.

Discussion

Our study indicated that the size of intimal entry zone strongly affects subsequent morphological differences. These results may serve as important clues to the mechanism of dissection, particularly aneurysm formation and dissecting occlusion. To induce morphological changes characteristic of dissection, a sufficiently large entry zone is needed. Most arteries with a short or intermediate longitudinal incision or a 2-mm elliptical endothelial defect (group I-A) eventually normalized. Such spontaneous healing due to shrinkage of the dissected pseudolumen might be possible because of limited extent and thickness of the subadventitial hematoma, which was too small to cause the stenotic change. Second, a medium-sized entry zone with a 4- or 6-mm long elliptical orifice (I-B or I-C) frequently resulted in saccular aneurysms corresponding to the site of intimal entry zone. This observation suggests that the size of entry zone is important for delayed aneurysm formation. Some reports describe the mechanism of saccular aneurysm dilation as hemodynamic stress that disrupts the intima, internal elastic lamina, and media at the entry point of arterial dissection

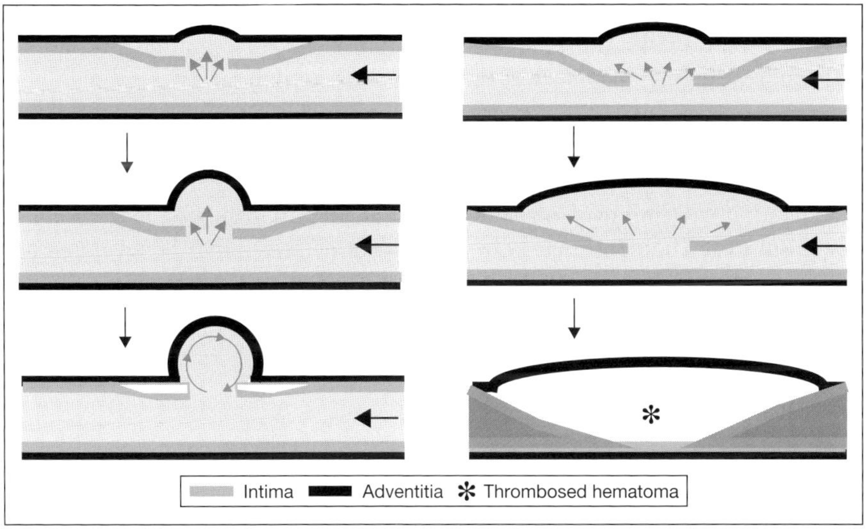

Fig. 5. Hypothesized schemes of aneurysm formation (left) and persistent stenosis (right). Hemodynamic stress from vortex flow inside the cavity may cause protrusion of the adventitia externally, resulting in a saccular aneurysm. However, a large entry zone can produce a massive, widespread subadventitial hematoma of sufficient size to compress the true lumen, resulting in abrupt occlusion. When the hematoma is large, the artery is likely to remain thrombosed.

[19]. We speculate that an unthrombosed dissected cavity can persist at the initial stage with a suitable balance of entering and exiting blood flow at the orifice [20–25]. At first a subadventitial hematoma may be only a diverticulum, but hemodynamic stress from vortex flow inside the cavity may cause further external protrusion of the adventitia, producing a saccular aneurysm (fig. 5).

Histopathologically, the dome of the aneurysm consisted of a layer of adventitia lined by newly formed endothelium. Such lack of a media containing smooth muscle is similar to the characteristics of intracranial aneurysms [26–30]. Thus, histopathological and macroscopic features of this experimental aneurysm approximate those of clinically encountered aneurysms more closely than a previous model using a sutured venous pouch [31].

A large entry zone can permit formation of a massive, extensive subadventitial hematoma sufficient to compress the true lumen, resulting in abrupt occlusion (fig. 5). When the hematoma is particularly large, the artery would be expected to remain thrombosed. However, some lesions with initial occlusion recanalized during the early period, probably because of vascular remodeling or distal migration of clots. The migration phenomenon may explain clinical episodes of distal intracranial embolism observed in the acute stage of cervical arterial dissection [4]. Thus, the most important factor determining morphological features and their course over time after dissection may be the extent of intimal injury irrespective of dissected layers.

Although our model is a traumatic dissection, a model of spontaneous dissection might be created by biochemical or molecular methods. Such further investigation will improve understanding of aneurysm formation in a variety of circumstances. The contribution of hemodynamic stress will be an important factor to assess in such experimental systems.

Conclusion

Morphological changes following experimental carotid dissection are affected by the size of the intimal entry zone. Very small dissections result in spontaneous healing, while large intimal entry zone cause stenotic lesions. However, a medium-sized entry zone (4–6 mm) may induce aneurysm formation. The different features of dissection may be caused by characteristics of flow into the subadventitial cavity and by thrombogenesis.

Consideration of intimal entry zone size is important for understanding the features of traumatic dissection of extracranial arteries, and experiments evaluating additional factors are needed to elucidate mechanisms of idiopathic and hypertensive arterial dissection.

References

1 Miyachi S, Ishiguchi T, Taniguchi K, Miyazaki M, Maeda K: Endovascular stenting of a traumatic dissecting aneurysm of the extracranial internal carotid artery. Neurol Med Chir (Tokyo) 1997;37: 270–274.

2 Fabian TC, George SM, Croce MA, Mangiante EC, Voeller GR, Kudsk KA: Carotid artery trauma: Management based on mechanism of injury. J Trauma 1990;30:953–963.

3 Mokri B, Piepgras G, Houser W: Traumatic dissection of the extracranial internal carotid artery. J Neurosurg 1988;68:189–197.

4 Pozzati E, Giuliani G, Poppi M, Faenza A: Blunt traumatic carotid dissection with delayed symptoms. Stroke 1989;20:412–416.

5 Miyachi S, Okamura K, Watanabe M, Inoue N, Nagatani T, Takagi T: Cerebellar stroke due to vertebral artery occlusion after cervical spine trauma. Spine 1994;19:83–88.

6 Hinse P, Thie A, Lachenmayer L: Dissection of the extracranial vertebral artery: Report of four cases and review of the literature. J Neurol Neurosurg Psychiatry 1991;54:863–869.

7 Mas JL, Bousser MG, Hasboun D, Laplane D: Extracranial vertebral artery dissections: A review of 13 cases. Stroke 1987;18:1037–1047.

8 Okada Y, Shima T, Nishida M, Yamane K, Kagawa R: Traumatic dissection of the common carotid artery after blunt injury to the neck. Surg Neurol 1999;51:513–520.

9 Ballard JL, Bunt TJ, Fitzpatrick B, Malone JM: Bilateral traumatic internal carotid artery dissections: Case report. J Vasc Surg 1992;15:431–435.

10 Anson J, Crowell RM: Cervicocranial arterial dissection. Neurosurgery 1991;29:89–96.
11 Stringer WL, Kelly DL: Traumatic dissection of the extracranial internal carotid artery. Neurosurgery 1980;6:123–130.
12 Hugenholtz H, Pokrupa R, Montpetit VJ, Nelson R, Richard MT: Spontaneous dissecting aneurysm of the extracranial vertebral artery. Neurosurgery 1982;10:96–100.
13 Kitanaka C, Tanaki J, Kuwahara M, Teraoka A, Sasaki T, Takakura K: Nonsurgical treatment of unruptured intracranial vertebral artery dissection with serial follow-up angiography. J Neurosurg 1994;80:667–674.
14 Okamoto T, Miyachi S, Negoro M, Otsuka G, Suzuki O, Keino H, Yoshida J: Experimental model of dissecting aneurysms. AJNR Am J Neuroradiol 2002;23:577–584.
15 Wilens SL, Malcolm JA, Vazquez JM: Experimental infarction (medical necrosis) of the dog's aorta. Am J Pathol 1965;47:695–711.
16 Takeoka T: An experimental study on dissecting aortic aneurysm (in Japanese). Journal of the Japanese Association for Thoracic Surgery 1984;32:174–186.
17 Farrell MA, Gilbert JJ, Kaufmann JC: Fatal intracranial arterial dissection: Clinical pathological correlation. J Neurol Neurosurg Psychiatry 1985;48:111–121.
18 Mizutani T, Miki Y, Kojima H, Suzuki H: Proposed classification of nonatherosclerotic cerebral fusiform and dissecting aneurysm. Neurosurgery 1999;45:253–260.
19 Takagi M, Hirata K, Fujitsu K, Yamamoto I: Unusual angiographic changes in a dissecting aneurysm of the basilar artery: Case report. Neurosurgery 1994;34:356–358.
20 Burleson AC, Strother CM, Turitto VT: Computer modeling of intracranial saccular and lateral aneurysms for the study of their hemodynamics. Neurosurgery 1995;37:774–784.
21 Gonzalez CF, Cho YI, Ortega HV, Moret J: Intracranial aneurysms: Flow analysis of their origin and progression. AJNR Am J Neuroradiol 1992;13:181–188.
22 Graves VB, Strother CM, Partington CR, Rappe A: Flow dynamics of lateral carotid artery aneurysms and their effects on coils and balloons: An experimental study in dogs. AJNR Am J Neuroradiol 1992;13:189–196.
23 Liepsch DW, Steiger HJ, Poll A, Reulen HJ: Hemodynamic stress in lateral saccular aneurysms. Biorheology 1987;24:689–710.
24 Perktold K, Gruber K, Kenner T, Florian H: Calculation of pulsatile flow and particle paths in an aneurysm-model. Basic Res Cardiol 1984;79:253–261.
25 Strother CM, Graves VB, Rappe A: Aneurysm hemodynamics: An experimental study. AJNR Am J Neuroradiol 1992;13:1089–1095.
26 Anidjar S, Salzmann JL, Gentric D, Lagneau P, Camilleri JP, Michel JB: Elastase-induced experimental aneurysms in rats. Circulation 1990;82:973–981.
27 Cawley CM, Dawson RC, Shengelaia G, Bonner G, Barrow DL, Colohan AR: Arterial saccular aneurysm model in the rabbit. AJNR Am J Neuroradiol 1996;17;1761–1766.
28 Halpern VJ, Nackman GB, Gandhi RH, Irizarry E, Scholes JV, Ramey WG, Tilson MD: The elastase infusion model of experimental aortic aneurysms: Synchrony of induction of endogenous proteinases with matrix destruction and inflammatory cell response. J Vasc Surg 1994;20: 51–60.
29 Kim C, Cervos-Navarro J, Kikuchi H, Hashimoto N, Hazama F: Degenerative changes in the internal elastic lamina relating to the development of saccular cerebral aneurysms in rats. Acta Neurochir (Wien) 1993;121:76–81.
30 Miskolczi L, Guterman LR, Flaherty JD, Hopkins LN: Saccular aneurysm induction by elastase digestion of the arterial wall: A new animal model. Neurosurgery 1998;43:595–601.
31 Varsos V, Heros RC, Debrun G, Zervas NT: Construction of experimental 'giant' aneurysms. Surg Neurol 1984;22:17–20.

Takeshi Okamoto, MD
Department of Neurosurgery
Nagoya University Graduate School of Medicine
65 Tsurumai-cho, Showa-ku, Nagoya-city, 466–8550 (Japan)
Tel. +81 52 744 2353, Fax +81 52 744 2360

Baumgartner RW, Bogousslavsky J, Caso V, Paciaroni M (eds): Handbook on Cerebral Artery Dissection. Front Neurol Neurosci. Basel, Karger, 2005, vol 20, pp 12–15

Epidemiology of Cervical Artery Dissection

Wouter I. Schievink, Vladimir Roiter

Maxine Dunitz Neurosurgical Institute and Department of Neurology, Cedars-Sinai Medical Center, Los Angeles, Calif., USA

Abstract

The diagnosis of cervical artery dissection has become routine. In young patients, spontaneous CAD is the cause of up to one-fourth of strokes. The incidence of spontaneous CAD is approximately 5 per 100,000 per year and is highest in autumn. The long-term recurrence rate is only approximately 1% per year, but it is higher in patients with familial arterial disease.

Not too long ago a patient with a spontaneous dissection of the extracranial carotid or vertebral artery was considered rare and the treatment of such a patient was a cause of considerable uncertainty. Nowadays, however, the diagnosis of spontaneous cervical artery dissection (CAD) has become routine largely due to the dramatic improvement of medical imaging and due to the growing awareness of CADs among healthcare professionals in the community. In studies performed in the 1980s, spontaneous CAD was found to be the cause in approximately 10–20% of young and middle-aged adults with ischemic stroke [1, 2]. In the late 1990s, this number increased to approximately 25% [3]. Spontaneous CAD can be considered to be one of the leading causes of stroke in the young and middle-aged population [4]. With aging, many additional risk factors contribute to stroke and thus spontaneous CAD accounts for only about 2–3% of all ischemic strokes among the elderly. Recent data, however, suggests that spontaneous CADs are underdiagnosed in the elderly [5]. The individual risk for a spontaneous CAD appears to be fairly equal over a person's life span, but it is slightly increased through the fifth decade of life [6]. Spontaneous CAD are equally common among the sexes and the only found sex predilection of arterial dissection is that it occurs approximately 5 years earlier in women than it does in men [6].

Incidence

In a retrospective community-based study in Rochester, Minnesota, we identified all patients diagnosed with spontaneous CAD from 1987 to 1992. The average annual incidence rate for all ages was 2.6 per 100,000 population [7]. Another community-based study conducted in France found a very similar rate for spontaneous internal carotid artery dissection of 3 per 100,000 per year [8]. We have previously estimated that the annual rate of vertebral artery dissection is approximately 1.5 per 100,000 per year [9]. Based on this data, the annual incidence rate of spontaneous CAD can be outlined as approximately 5 per 100,000 [9]. In a recent Emergency-Department-based series (2003–2004), we identified 7 patients with spontaneous carotid artery dissection compared to 12 with spontaneous subarachnoid hemorrhage, for an estimated incidence of approximately 5 per 100,000 [Schievink et al., unpubl. data].

It has been shown that the frequency of spontaneous CAD is higher in autumn than in other seasons [10]. The exact reason for this seasonal variation is unclear, but it may be related to a higher frequency of certain infectious diseases, which may precipitate the occurrence of spontaneous carotid artery dissection.

Recurrence

Among patients with spontaneous CAD, the risk of a recurrent arterial dissection was investigated in several studies. Schievink et al. [6] conducted a study among 200 consecutive patients with spontaneous CAD. During an average follow-up of 7.4 years, 16 patients (8%) had a recurrent arterial dissection. Approximately one-fourth of patients suffered from multivessel disease. The highest rate of recurrence (2%) was shown within the first month after the initial event. The reported cumulative rate of a recurrent dissection among patients followed for 10 years was approximately 12%. Given the fact that recurrent dissections occurred only in arteries not previously involved by dissection, it may be postulated that an acute phase exists of an underlying arterial wall disease predisposing to the occurrence of a dissection. In a study reported by Leys et al. [11], a recurrence of CAD was found in 3 (3%) of 105 patients during an average follow-up of 36 months. Similar results were obtained by Bassetti et al. [12]. In their study, 4% out of 81 patients had a recurrent internal CAD during a 4-year follow-up. The average risk of a recurrent CAD can be estimated at a relatively low 1% per year, although patients with a family history of arterial dissection probably have a considerably higher risk [13]. Two hundred patients with a diagnosis of spontaneous CAD were included in the study of Schievink et al. [6]. A recurrent arterial dissection was identified in

50% of patients with familial arterial disease compared with only 6% of patients with non-familial disease. The estimated relative risk was 6.3. Therefore, it can be concluded that a family history of arterial dissection is an important risk factor for the development of a recurrent artery dissection.

'Provoked' CAD

A history of a more or less trivial precipitating event is a frequent finding in patients with CAD. The mechanisms and the severity of trauma vary widely from penetrating neck injury or severe motor-vehicle-crash-related injury to very minor movements of the neck. It is been established for a long time that cervical chiropractic and osteopathic procedures may have serious neurological consequences, including CAD. Such manipulations have recently become more recognized by neurologists as a potential cause of vertebral artery and even internal artery dissections, whereas most practitioners of spinal manipulation are of the opinion that these events are extremely rare [14]. Such an obvious referral bias was clearly encountered in the study of Haldeman et al. [15] based on chiropractic reports. The estimated rate of vertebral artery dissection was reported as one in almost 6 million cervical manipulations. The fact that a patient who has a stroke will likely be seen by only one chiropractor but by three or more neurologists may explain at least in part the difference in experience and the perception of risks among these two professions. A wide range anywhere between 1 in 20,000 to 1 in 1 million of potentially harmful complications of cervical spine manipulation has been reported [16]. The true frequency of CAD associated with chiropractic manipulation of the spine remains obscure. Given the real, albeit low, risk of cervical manipulation, it should only be performed in patients without predisposing factors for artery dissection, with fully informed consent by the patient, and after an appropriate diagnosis of neck pain. In one study, we found that a large number of patients with CAD associated with chiropractic manipulation of the spine either had an obvious generalized arteriopathy, a likely diagnosis of vertebral artery dissection prior to the neck manipulation, or both [17].

References

1 Bogousslavsky J, Despland PA, Regli F: Spontaneous carotid dissection with acute stroke. Arch Neurol 1987;44:137–140.

2 Cronqvist SE, Norrving B, Nilsson B: Young stroke patients: An angiographic study. Acta Radiol 1986; 369(suppl):34–37.

3 Ducrocq X, Lacour JC, Debouverie M, Bracard S, Girard F, Weber M: Accidents vasculaires cerebraux ischémiques du sujet jeune: étude prospective de 296 patients ages de 16 a 45 ans. Rev Neurol 1999;155:575–582.

4 Schievink WI, Mokri B, Piepgras DG: Spontaneous dissections of cervicocephalic arteries in childhood and adolescence. Neurology 1994;44:1607–1612.
5 Ahl B, Bokemeyer M, Ennen JC, Kohlmetz C, Becker H, Weissenborn K: Dissection of the brain supplying arteries over the life span. J Neurol Neurosurg Psychiatry 2004;74:1194–1196.
6 Schievink WI, Mokri B, O'Fallon WM: Recurrent spontaneous cervical artery dissection. N Engl J Med 1994;330:393–397.
7 Schievink WI, Mokri B, Whisnant JP: Internal carotid artery dissection in a community. Stroke 1993;24:1678–1680.
8 Giroud M, Fayolle H, Andre N, Dumas R, Becker F, Martin D, Baudoin N, Krause D: Incidence of internal carotid artery dissection in the community of Dijon. J Neurol Neurosurg Psychiatry 1994;57:1443.
9 Schievink WI: Spontaneous dissection of the carotid and vertebral arteries. N Engl J Med 2001;344.899–906.
10 Schievink WI, Wijdicks EFM, Kuiper JD: Seasonal pattern of spontaneous cervical artery dissection. J Neurosurg 1998;89:101–103.
11 Leys D, Moulin T, Stoijkovic T, Begey S, Chavot D, DONALD Investigators: Follow-up of patients with history of cervical artery dissection. Cerebrovasc Dis 1995;5:43–49.
12 Bassetti C, Carruzzo A, Sturzenegger M, Tuncdogan E: Recurrence of cervical artery dissection. Stroke 1996;27:1804–1807.
13 Schievink WI, Mokri B, Piepgras DG, Kuiper JD: Recurrent spontaneous arterial dissections: Risk in familial versus nonfamilial disease. Stroke 1996;27:622–624.
14 Hufnagel A, Hammers A, Schonle PW, Bohm KD, Leonhardt G: Stroke following chiropractic manipulation of the cervical spine. J Neurol 1999;246:683–688.
15 Haldeman S, Kohlbeck FJ, McGregor M: Risk factors and precipitating neck movements causing vertebrobasilar dissection after cervical trauma and spinal manipulation. Spine 1999;24:785–794.
16 Vickers A, Zollman C: ABC of complementary medicine. The manipulative therapies: Osteopathy and chiropractic. Br Med J 1999;319:1176–1179.
17 Schievink WI, Mokri B, Piepgras D, Parisi J, Silbert P: Cervical artery dissections assoicated with chiropractic manipulation of the neck. The importance of pre-existing arterial disease and injury (abstract). J Neurol 1996;243(suppl.2):S92.

Wouter I. Schievink, MD
Maxine Dunitz Neurosurgical Institute and Department of Neurology
Cedars-Sinai Medical Center, 8631 W 3rd Street, #800-E
Los Angeles, CA 90048 (USA)
Tel. +1 310 423 7900, Fax +1 310 423 0810, E-Mail schievinkw@cshs.org

Baumgartner RW, Bogousslavsky J, Caso V, Paciaroni M (eds): Handbook on Cerebral Artery Dissection. Front Neurol Neurosci. Basel, Karger, 2005, vol 20, pp 16–29

Association of Cervical Artery Dissection with Connective Tissue Abnormalities in Skin and Arteries

T. Brandt[a,b], *M. Morcher*[b], *I. Hausser*[c]

[a]Kliniken Schmieder Heidelberg, [b]Department of Neurology,
[c]Department of Dermatology, University of Heidelberg, Heidelberg, Germany

Abstract

Spontaneous cervical artery dissections (sCAD) often occur in otherwise healthy individuals without known risk factors for stroke and frequently develop spontaneously without relevant trauma. An underlying arteriopathy leading to a so-called 'weakness of the vessel wall' and predisposing certain individuals to dissection has often been postulated. Therefore, the morphology of connective tissue, a main component of vessel wall and environment, was investigated in carotids and skin. While the overall morphology of dermal connective tissue is normal, about half of patients with sCAD show mild ultrastructural connective tissue alterations. These ultrastructural morphological aberrations can be designated either as 'Ehlers-Danlos syndrome (EDS) III-like', resembling mild findings in patients with the hypermobility type of EDS (EDS III); or coined 'EDS IV-like' with collagen fibers containing fibrils with highly variable diameters resembling mild findings in vascular EDS; or the abnormalities are restricted to the elastic fibers (with fragmentation and minicalcifications) without significant alterations in the morphology of the collagen fibrils. These findings had some similarity with the morphology found in heterozygous carriers of pseudoxanthoma elasticum. A grading scale according to the severity of the findings has been introduced. Similar connective tissue abnormalities were detected in some first-degree relatives of patients with sCAD showing hereditary at least in a subgroup. They can serve as a phenotypic marker for further genetic studies in patients with sCAD and large families to possibly identify the underlying basic molecular defect(s). Very few of patients (<5%) with sCAD and connective tissue abnormalities have clinical manifestations of skin, joint, or skeletal abnormalities of a defined heritable connective tissue disorder. In specimens of arterial walls of carotid, aortic, and renal arteries of patients with sCAD, pronounced systemic, histopathological, and ultrastructural abnormalities were detected with elastic fiber fragmentation and medial degeneration, described before only in a few patients with known hereditary connective tissue diseases such as the Marfan syndrome. We hypothesize that a major part of sCAD cases represents a manifestation of a connective tissue disorder with a vascular phenotype.

Dissection often occurs in otherwise healthy individuals without known risk factors for stroke and frequently develops spontaneously without relevant trauma [1, 2]. The question has been posed why a dissection happens in certain individuals, in some possibly triggered by a common daily life movement stretching a cervical artery while in most individuals nothing ever occurs – even very infrequently with a severe head trauma [3]. An underlying arteriopathy leading to a so-called 'weakness of the vessel wall' and predisposing to dissection has often been postulated in spontaneous cervical artery dissections (sCAD), particularly because frequently more than one cervico-cerebral vessel is involved and patients are often of a younger age [1, 4]. The high prevalence of sCAD in patients with fibromuscular dysplasia and hereditary connective tissue disorders, such as the Ehlers-Danlos syndrome (EDS), also suggests the involvement of vessel wall abnormalities [5, 6]. An impairment of the vessel wall may be correlated with alterations of their extracellular matrix environment, which may be caused by systemic connective tissue component aberrations [4, 7]. As endarterectomy is usually not used to treat sCAD and postmortem examinations are rare, histomorphological examination of the dissected vessel wall, however, is seldom performed. Therefore, the skin might serve as a so-called 'window', as an indirect approach to possible connective tissue abnormalities of the arterial walls [7]. Similarly, ultrastructural analysis of dermal connective tissue serves as a routine diagnostic tool in patients at risk for many types of connective tissue disorders, e.g., cutis laxa, pseudoxanthoma elasticum (PXE), or EDS [7–10], since a definite molecular genetic diagnosis has not been established.

Recently, connective tissue aberrations were shown for the first time to correlate, indeed frequently, with sCAD in otherwise healthy individuals [4, 11]. In a multicenter study we further analyzed the association of sCAD with ultrastructural abnormalities of the dermal connective tissue in another, larger series of patients from different centers [12]. Follow-up biospies in some patients addressed the question of intraindividual variability of the findings over time [11].

Moreover, we found in specimens of arterial walls of carotid, aortic, and renal arteries of patients with sCAD pronounced systemic histopathological and ultrastructural abnormalities, described before only in a few patients with known hereditary connective tissue diseases such as the Marfan syndrome [13]. We hypothesize that a major part of sCAD cases represents a manifestation of a genetic predisposition with a vascular phenotype. Ultrastructural dermal connective tissue abnormalities could be a further phenotypic marker in those patients and be used for familial genetic studies in the future to possibly identify the underlying molecular defect(s).

In this chapter we also describe the technical handling and the diagnostic evaluation of skin biopsies in order to standardize the assessment of the delicate morphological abnormalities that are usually found in patients with sCAD.

Preparations for Light and Electron Microscopy

Skin biopsies are taken from the outer aspect of the upper arm close (about 10 cm) to the elbow [7–10]. The skin is thoroughly and repeatedly sterilized with 70% ethanol. An almond-shaped piece of skin (10 × 5 mm) is excised with vertical deep knife incisions extending into the subcutaneous fat tissue. The biopsy sample is subsequently cut into two pieces. One part is processed for transmission electron microscopy, the other part is immediately processed for tissue culturing of fibroblasts. Squashing of the excised piece of skin, either during excision, or during the handling with the forceps must be carefully avoided, as additional mechanical stress might be a possible source of morphological artifacts.

The artery specimens were taken during surgery or postmortem.

Biopsy specimens are initially fixed in 3% glutaraldehyde in 0.1 *M* Na-cacodylate buffer (pH 7.4) at room temperature, cut into pieces of approximately 1 mm^3 and fixed in the same solution for some more hours. After being washed in buffer solution, specimens were postfixed in 1% OsO_4 in 0.1 *M* Na-cacodylate buffer (pH 7.4), rinsed in water, passed through a graded ethanol dehydration series, transferred to propylene oxide, embedded in epoxy resin (glycidether 100 or Epon 812) and cut after completed polymerization into semithin and ultrathin sections. Semithin sections are stained with methylene blue and evaluated by light microscopy. It has to be carefully documented which part of the skin (upper, middle, and deep dermis) or the arterial wall (intima, media, adventitia) was to be cut into ultrathin sections. Ultrathin sections are treated with uranyl acetate, contrasted with lead citrate and examined with a Philips EM 400 transmission electron microscope.

Morphology of Dermal Connective Tissue

On the light microscopical level, the dermal connective tisssue did not reveal regular pathological alterations. The ultrastructural aspect of connective tissue components, i.e., collagen fibrils and elastic fibers, is to be investigated for in all regions of the skin of each patient [7–10]. The findings are to be compared with those of age-matched controls with stroke of other origins. We also used a large number of other control samples available from the skin biopsy bank of the Electron Microscopic Laboratory, Department of Dermatology, Heidelberg (more than 5,000 patients included so far). For morphological differences, the focus is on the reticular dermal region, where connective tissue structures are usually very regular and not affected by environmental factors,

Table 1. Grading of ultrastructural connective tissue abnormalities

Collagen fibril abnormalities
–Mild aberrations (+)
Regular irregularities of the contours and calibers of the collagen fibrils with only few single composite collagen fibrils within collagen bundles
–Pronounced aberrations (++)
More frequent irregularities of the contours and calibers of the collagen fibrils with more frequent but still single composite collagen fibrils
–Severe aberrations (+++)
Anomalies with frequent composite, flower-like fibrils in many collagen bundles, degree of severity of collagen fiber aberrations comparable with EDS III
Elastic fiber abnormalities
–Mild aberrations (+)
Regular but mild irregularities of the contours of the elastic fibers. Only few electron-dense inclusions (microcalcifications)
–Pronounced aberrations (++)
Frequent irregularities of the contours of the elastic fibers, reaching in some fibers a fragmented 'moth-eaten' aspect; several electron-dense inclusions (microcalcifications)
–Severe aberrations (+++)
Frequent fragmented elastic fibers, reaching a degree of severity a 'moth-eaten' porous aspect, resembling the findings of the marfanoid hypermobility syndrome; frequent electron-dense inclusions (microcalcifications)
Findings of the deep skin layers of the reticular dermis to exclude degenerative changes as e.g. actinic elastosis

for instance actinic elastosis. For the severity of the connective tissue aberrations a semiquantitative classification was introduced earlier (table 1). We consider abnormalities as 'marked' with at least a '2 plus'-severity on the scale as defined. All other pathological findings are classified as 'mild'. Others, including borderline findings not definitely meeting these criteria, are considered as 'normal'. The structure of the collagen fibrils (in cross-section) and the elastic fibers should also be studied at high magnifications (>10,000×) in order to detect typical aberrations like composite collagen fibrils or minicalcifications in the elastic material. Experience with skin samples from patients with known inherited connective tissue disorders, notably with several subtypes of EDS, is helpful for the classification of the skin samples from patients with sCAD, since most abnormalities in sCAD patients range in severity and aspect somewhere between normality and those in patients with EDS [7–10].

Table 2. Electron microscopic analysis of 126 skin biopsies of patients with spontaneous cervical artery dissections (sCAD)

Type of dissections	EDS-III-like	EDS-IV-like	Only elastic fibers	Normal
sCAD of single vessel	33	7	11	36
sCAD of multiple vessels	10	6	5	18

The electron microscopic findings were classified as 'EDS-III-like', 'EDS-IV-like' or 'only elastic fibers'. In the families of 10 patients with sCAD a first-degree relative also had a history of sCAD. EDS = Ehlers-Danlos syndrome. The group of patients with sCAD of multiple vessels consists of patients with recurrent dissections as well as patients with multiple simultaneous dissections.

If clinical and laboratory data suggest the presence of a known connective tissue disorder, in some cases complementary molecular genetic tests, e.g. for the vascular EDS with COL3A1, can be made to confirm the diagnosis [12, 13].

Skin biopsies from 126 patients with sCAD and from 29 healthy relatives were investigated so far [14]. Six specimens could not be evaluated, due to artificial modifications of the morphology caused by improper handling (2 biopsies were not deep enough, 1 consisted only of fat, 1 was squashed too strongly, and 2 were damaged during transport because the tube with fixation solution was leaking). The quality of 149 out of 155 biopsies (96%) was good enough for a reliable histological and electron microscopic analysis.

In 72 biopsies from patients with sCAD we found morphological aberrations but only on the electron microscopic level (fig. 1, 2). On the basis of the morphology we classified the aberrations into 3 groups (tables 1, 2). Within each group the aberrations varied in strength (in quantity). In a previous study of skin biopsies from patients with intracranial aneurysms, we differentiated between aberrations of a EDS-III-like pattern and those of a EDS-IV-like pattern. In those cases the morphology had similarities with the findings in patients with EDS-III or EDS-IV, although the structural abnormalities in patients with EDS-III and EDS-IV are usually more dramatic than those in patients with aneurysms only [17]. In our series of patients with sCAD we again detected both types of connective tissue aberrations. Moreover, we discerned a third group of patients with aberrations restricted to the elastic fiber system resembling the findings of heterozygote carriers of recessive PXE (PXE-carrier-like) [16].

All 8 patients in whom a second biopsy was performed showed identical ultrastructural findings and were ranked at the same level of pathomorphological

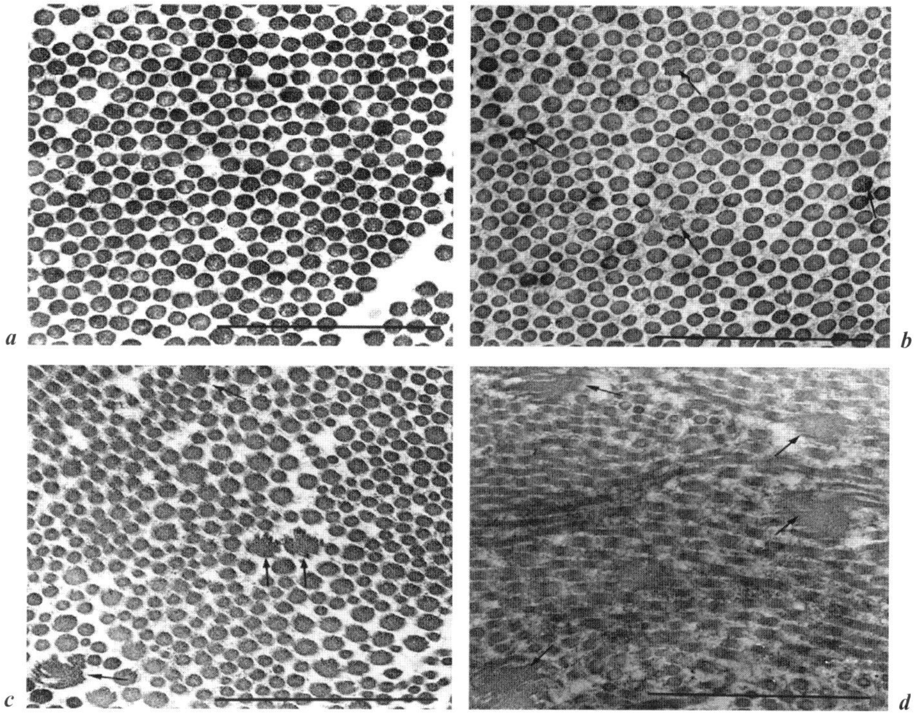

Fig. 1. ***a*** Normal collagen bundles within reticular dermis consist of large, densely packed collagen fibrils with uniform cross-sections (control); electron microscopy (EM) ×43,000. ***b, c*** Collagen aberrations in 2 patients with spontaneous arterial dissection. ***b*** Mild aberrations ('+' according to table 1) consisting of collagen bundles within the reticular dermis containing single or several fibrils with irregular contours and composite (flower-like) fibrils (arrows); the calibers of the aberrant fibrils vary; EM ×43,000. ***c*** Severe aberrations ('+++' according to table 1), including numerous composite fibrils (arrows), within the mid-dermal collagen bundles and enlarged diameters of the composite fibrils; EM ×43,000. ***d*** Collagen aberrations in a patient with spontaneous arterial dissection and minor stigmata of EDS II (small pseudomolluscoid scars at elbows): Collagen bundles within the reticular dermis contain frequent composite (flower-like) fibrils (arrows); EM ×31,000. Bars correspond to 1 μm each.

severity in both analyses [11]. In the 6 cases with familial sCAD, similar findings were seen: 4 had mild aberrations (EDS IV-like in 2), and 2 did not have any distinct pathological findings [14]. Connective tissue abnormalities were not found more frequently in patients with multivessel sCAD. Connective tissue aberrations were more frequently found in male patients with sCAD than in female patients, and were associated with recurrent sCAD, but not with age and vascular risk factors [11].

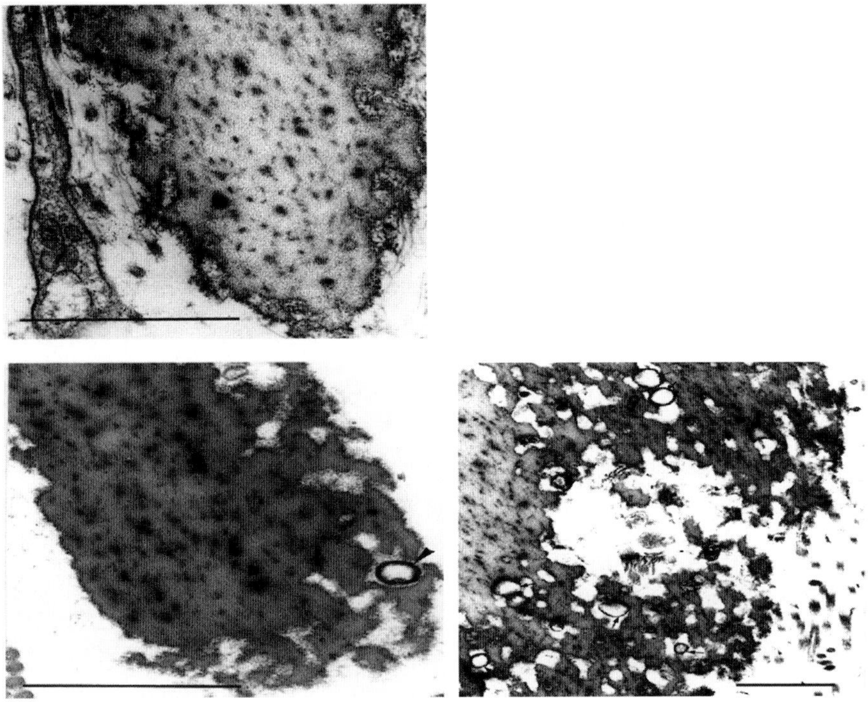

a b c

Fig. 2. ***a*** Normal mature elastic fiber in the reticular dermis presents with an amorphous elastin core surrounded by elastotubules (control); EM ×26,000. ***b, c*** Elastic fiber aberrations in 2 patients with spontaneous arterial dissection. ***b*** Regular but mild irregularities of the contours of the elastic fibers, focal electron-dense deposit (arrowhead) ('+' according to table 1); EM ×20,000. ***c*** Focal electron-dense deposits representing minicalcifications (arrows) and pronounced fragmentation with a moth-eaten, porous aspect ('+++' according to table 1); EM ×9,000. Arterial ultrastructural connective tissue findings in patients with sCAD and controls. Bars correspond to 1 μm each.

Only 3 patients of our series (<5%) presented with clinical signs of a connective tissue disorder with hyperextensible skin and joints in 1, a marfanoid appearance in another, and hypertrophic pseudomolluscoid scars at the elbows in a 3rd patient. Another patient had a history of 4 spontaneous abortions.

For the light and electron microscopic examination of diagnostic skin biopsies, the findings in patients must be compared to findings in healthy control subjects. The distinction between normal and abnormal morphology might be difficult in some cases, as there is a smooth transition from perfectly normal into definitely abnormal. A connective tissue diagnosis can therefore rarely be made on the sole basis of isolated electron micrographs of a single patient. The assessment of the morphology depends as a rule on a variety of clinical, histological and electron microscopic observations, as well as on extended experience with other patients and with control subjects. We classified the ultrastructural alterations in skin biopsies from patients into three different groups, which are compared to the findings in patients with known connective tissue disorders [14]. In an earlier analysis of the ELN gene in patients with sCAD we had already alluded to a possible differentiation between patterns of aberrant morphology and included some patients with aberrations only in the elastic fibers [12]. A subsequent study of connective tissue in patients with intracranial aneurysms obviously revealed the existence of two different types of morphological alterations [17]. Our findings confirm the morphological heterogeneity in a large series of sCAD patients and the existence of different classes of aberrations with quantitative differences within each class. The analogy with the findings in patients with EDS III and EDS IV [10] and in heterozygous PXE [8, 9] carriers suggests that genetic heterogeneity exists amongst patients with sCAD. In previous work we [4, 15] showed various electron micrographs of EDS-III-like connective tissue aberrations, the most common type found amongst patients with sCAD.

The ultrastructural dermal findings, however, are not specific for any distinct connective tissue disorder or genetic defect [7–10]. Further quantitative morphometric analysis of these findings might be helpful, but to our knowledge is not used for diagnostic EM in connective tissue disorders at present. Qualitatively similar deviations may be seen in patients with various heritable connective tissue diseases, i.e., composite collagen fibrils in patients with EDS, osteogenesis imperfecta type I, and PXE [7–10], and are also found in some acquired conditions but in restricted areas only (e.g., lymphedema or rheumatoid arthritis) [7–10]. Fragmented elastic fibers with focal osmiophilic deposits are found in patients with PXE, Marfan syndrome, and marfanoid hypermobility syndrome, as well as in patients with severe EDS types I and II [7–10]. It is the specific pattern of structural deviations that characterizes a connective tissue disorder [7–10]. The overall pattern and combination of the ultrastructural aberrations of collagen and elastic material, combined with the clinical phenotype of the patients with sCAD investigated, are unique and not yet known for a defined heritable connective tissue disorder. In some of the patients the pronounced ultrastructural aberrations with frequent composite collagen fibrils resemble those found in EDS type III or even II; however, differing clinical features with vascular manifestation and lack of phenotypic signs of these types of EDS point to a distinct connective tissue disorder of a yet unknown nature. Whether this is a new disease entity or just a minor variant of a known connective tissue disorder is speculative. Strikingly, similar morphological changes were detected recently in healthy heterozygote carriers in families with recessive PXE [16].

Hints for the Hereditary of the Morphological Alterations

The segregation of the connective tissue alterations was analyzed in 4 pedigrees. In 3 families we observed EDS-III-like connective tissue aberrations (fig. 1a–c) [14, 18]. From these families we analyzed 21 individuals. The 3 index patients and 9 healthy relatives displayed similar aberrations, 8 further healthy relatives did not show connective tissue alterations, and in 1 of the relatives the aberrations were much weaker than in the index patient. The 1:1 ratio of carriers and noncarriers as well as the segregation patterns within the families suggest an autosomal dominant inheritance. The segregation in the family of the patient with EDS-IV-like aberrations seems to be different. The segregation pattern is compatible both with an autosomal dominant and with a recessive mode of inheritance. However, it is also possible that the connective tissue alterations in this family are not inherited at all. We moreover observed very weak connective tissue aberrations in both sons of a sister without connective tissue phenotype. A further investigation of the father of these both sons showed that the father did not carry a connective tissue phenotype.

The segregation analysis in three families suggested that the EDS-III-like alterations are inherited. Hence, these morphological connective tissue alterations were considered as a reliable subclinical phenotype and might be associated with an unknown mutation.

Morphology of Vessel Walls

Arterial wall specimens (internal carotid arteries in all, additionally aortic artery specimens in 3, renal in 2, and vertebral in 2) of 12 sCAD patients (3 postmortem and 9 during carotid endarterectomy) were investigated and compared to specimens of 7 age-matched control specimens (internal carotid artery from patients after nonvascular death) [15].

Correlation with dermal connective tissue could be performed in 5 patients, in 3 the arterial wall specimens showed much more pronounced findings in the elastic fibers in contrast to normal or very light findings in the dermal ultrastructure, and 2 had similar pathological alterations.

In contrast to dermal morphology, however, the vessel wall architecture was already altered on the light mircroscopical level. In normal specimens, the wall is built of regularly stratified layers encompassing the intima lined by the lamina elastica interna, the media with parallel elastic fibers and myocytes, and the adventitia containing more loosely packed collagen bundles and less elastic material. Ultrastructurally, the margin of the elastic fibers appears smooth.

In carotid walls of sCAD patients, the structure of the intima was often irregular with thickenings and interruptions. Within the media, most conspicuous was a disorganization of the parallel arrangement of elastic fibers, - vacuolization of myocytes, and overall fibrotic appearance. While already the first histopathological description of sCAD by Anderson and Schlechter [19] found a systemic arteriopathy with medial degeneration, in most reviews mostly normal histopathology findings were, probably without sufficient systematic data, assumed [3].

By electron microscopy, elastic fibers were fragmented in all arterial specimens of sCAD patients that we had investigated and it revealed highly inhomogeneous margins with irregular protrusions; in some regions elastic material was rarefied (fig. 3a, b, fig. 4a–d). Myocytes were often filled with empty irregular vacuoles and lipid droplets (fig. 3c, d).

The overall appearance of the pathological alterations on the histological and ultrastructural level is most similar to the so-called cystic medial degeneration [15, 19, 20]. This purely descriptive pathology is found in degenerative vascular disorders as well as in hereditary connective tissue diseases, such as the Marfan syndrome, with very few examinations, however, performed up to now for these entities [19, 20]. These constant findings of a systemic arteriopathy are a first evidence for the hypothesis of a generalized connective tissue disorder particularly affecting the vascular system predisposing otherwise healthy individuals to sCAD.

Phenotypic Expression

Similar to a vascular phenotype of PXE [16], the clinical manifestation of a connective tissue disorder might be limited to the vascular system as in our group of patients showing no external signs of a known connective tissue disease [5, 6]. Also, very subtle signs might only be recognized by experienced examiners. Indeed, one of our patients with sCAD who showed pronounced ultrastructural collagen fibril aberrations in the skin biopsy corresponding to EDS type II had only mild cardinal symptoms of EDS type II, with small hypertrophic pseudomolluscoid scars at the elbows. No other patient, except one with a marfanoid appearance and another with signs characteristic for EDS, showed external stigmata for a known connective tissue disorder. In a prospective series, in 3 of 15 patients (20%) with sCAD, phenotypic signs for a heritable connective tissue disease were found, such as a marfanoid appearance, hyperextensible skin with abnormal scars, joint hypermobility, or femoral hernia [16]. Further classification of these still unnamed disorders by biochemical studies for collagen I and III, and fibrillin-1 abnormalities, however, was

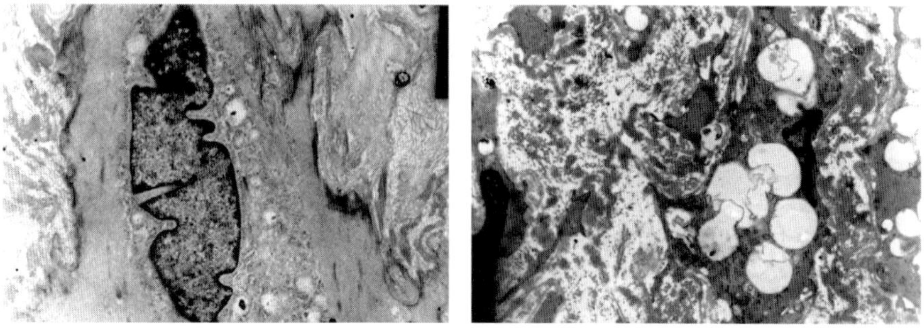

a *b*

Fig. 3. Cellular abnormalities. ***a*** Normal myocyte (internal carotid artery, medial layer); control (EM ×15,000). ***b*** Myocyte with pronounced vacuolization (internal carotid artery, medial layer); sCAD (EM ×12,000).

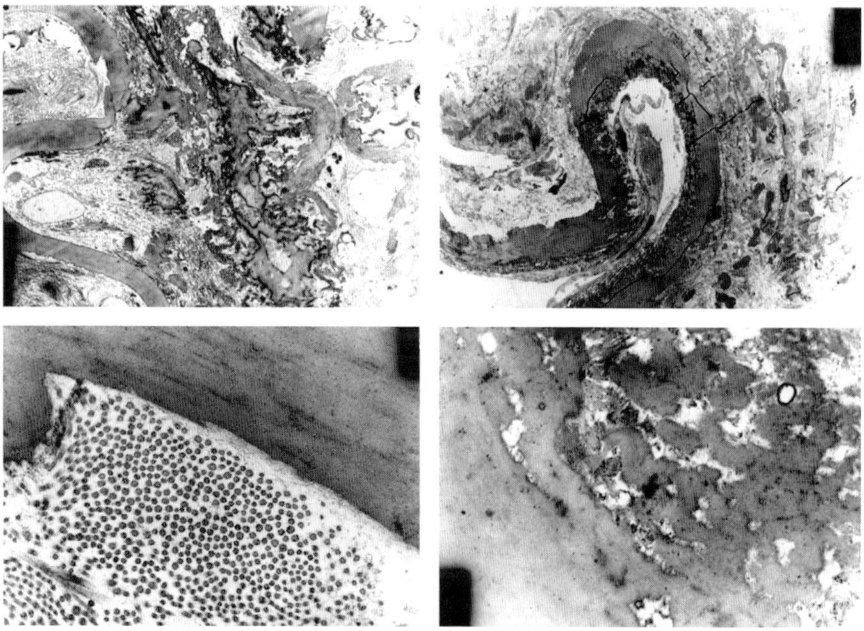

a *b* *c* *d*

Fig. 4. Elastic fiber aberrations. ***a*** Normal control with regular contour and content (internal carotid artery, medial layer; control, EM ×6,000). ***b*** Abnormal elastic fiber with irregular contour (sCAD; internal carotid artery, medial layer); sCAD (EM × 2,500). ***c*** High magnification of normal control with regular contour and content (internal carotid artery, medial layer); control (EM ×43,000). ***d*** Fragmentation with porous aspect and minicalcification in sCAD patient (internal carotid artery, medial layer; EM ×43,000).

unsuccessful. In another patient with sCAD and no phenotypic signs other than slightly bluish sclerae, a mutation characteristic of osteogenesis imperfecta type I was identified (see chapter by Grond-Ginsbach et al., pp. 30–43). Unfortunately, EM was not performed in either study.

Dissections and Connective Tissue Abnormalities

The pathogenesis of sCAD is still unclear [21]. The hypothesis of an underlying connective tissue disorder leading to a structural instability of the arterial wall is supported by the high incidence of dissections and cerebral aneurysms in patients with known heritable connective tissue disorders such as EDS type IV [4, 5, 21]. Half of all patients biopsied for the dermal ultrastructure showed aberrations of collagen fibrils and elastic fibers within the reticular dermis. Moreover, follow-up biopsies taken from a different location did not disclose intraindividual variability over time [11]. This suggests that the abnormalities in the dermal connective tissue represent a constant finding in these patients. Familial sCAD with connective tissue abnormalities showed a similar pathomorphology [18]. Furthermore, in addition to the patients with familial sCAD, we recently established identical connective tissue abnormalities in skin biopsies in 3 out of 4 so far unaffected children of a patient with sCAD who showed pronounced ultrastructural aberrations [18]. The obvious inheritance shown supports the hypothesis of a genetic origin of sCAD, at least in a subgroup of patients. Positive findings for ultrastructural connective tissue abnormalities were recently confirmed by two other groups for sCAD, one with 12 positive out of 22 (54%) patients, and the more recent one with 5 out of 6 patients having an 'EDS-like' dermal ultrastructure [22, 23]. As reported by the first authors, only 1 of the other 23 patients with traumatic CAD showed these aberrations on EM [22] indicating that there is likely to be a different pathogenesis for the two types of sCAD abnormalities.

As the mechanical stability and elasticity of the vessel wall is provided by connective tissue elements [7, 20] structural deviations in the main components, collagen and elastic fibers, may lead to functional impairment, predisposing to dissection of the arterial wall at given points of minor resistance. The regular presence of composite collagen fibrils and fragmented elastic fibers in patients with sCAD points to basic defects within the extracellular matrix [4, 7, 11, 20]. Ultrastructural studies in the cervical arteries of patients with sCAD correlate the dermal findings with the ultrastructure of the arterial walls [15]. In some the ultrastructure of the vessel is even more pronounced resembling findings of the so-called medial degeneration or necrosis. We speculate that many sCAD patients with negative skin biopsies possibly show connective tissue abnormalities in arterial specimens.

A combination of an underlying arteriopathy as genetic predisposition and temporarily active factors may be necessary for sCAD to occur at a certain point in time [21].

References

1 Hart RG, Easton JD: Dissections (editorial). Stroke 1985;16:925–927.

2 Norris JW, Beletsky V, Nadareishvili Z: 'Spontaneous' cervical arterial dissection. Stroke 2002; 33:1945–1946.

3 Schievink W: Spontaneous dissection of the carotid and vertebral arteries. N Engl J Med 2001; 344:898–906.

4 Brandt T, Hausser I, Orberk E, Grau A, Hartschuh W, Anton-Lamprecht I, Hacke W: Ultrastructural connective tissue abnormalities in patients with spontaneous cervicocerebral artery dissections. Ann Neurol 1998;44:281–285.

5 Pepin M, Schwarze U, Superti-Furga A, Byers PH: Clinical and genetic features of Ehlers-Danlos syndrome type IV, the vascular type. N Engl J Med 2000;342:673–680.

6 Schievink WI, Michels VV, Piepgras DG: Neurovascular manifestations of heritable connective tissue disorders (review). Stroke 1994;25:889–903.

7 Holbrook KA, Byers PH: Skin is a window on heritable disorders of connective tissue. Am J Med Genet 1989;34:105–121.

8 Anton-Lamprecht I: The skin; in Papadimitriou JM, Henderson DW, Spagnolo DV (eds): Diagnostic Ultrastructure of Non-Neoplastic Diseases. Edinburgh, Churchill Livingstone, 1992, pp 90–109.

9 Royce PM, Steinman B: Connective Tissue and Its Heritable Disorders. Molecular, Genetic, and Medical Aspects. New York, Wiley-Liss Inc., 1993.

10 Hausser I, Anton-Lamprecht I: Differential ultrastructural aberrations of collagen fibrils in Ehlers-Danlos syndrome types I-IV as a means for diagnostics and classification. Hum Genet 1994;93: 394–407.

11 Brandt T, Orberk E, Weber R, Werner I, Busse O, Muller BT, Wigger F, Grau A, Grond-Ginsbach C, Hausser I: Pathogenesis of cervical artery dissections: Association with connective tissue abnormalities. Neurology 2001;57:24–30.

12 Kuivaniemi H, Prockop DJ, Wu Y, Madhatheri SL, Kleinert C, Earley JJ, Jokinen A, Stolle C, Majamaa K, Myllyla VV, Norrgard O, Schievink WI, Mokri B, Fukawa O, ter Berg HWM, De Paepe A, Lozano AM, Leblanc R, Ryynanen M, Baxter BT, Shikata H, Ferell RE, Tromp G. Exclusion of mutations in the gene for type III collagen (COL3A1) as a common cause of intracranial aneurysms or cervical artery dissections: Results from sequence analysis of the coding sequences of type III collagen from 55 unrelated patients. Neurology 1993;43:2652–2658.

13 van den Berg JS, Limburg M, Kappelle LJ, Pals G, Arwert F, Westerveld A: The role of type III collagen in spontaneous cervical arterial dissections. Ann Neurol 1998;43:494–498.

14 Hausser I, Müller U, Entgelter S, Lyrer P, Pezzini A, Padovani A, Moormann B, Busse O, Weber R, Brandt T, Grond-Ginsbach C: Different types of connective tissue alterations associated with cervical artery dissections. Acta Neuropathol 2004;107:509–514.

15 Brandt T, Grond-Ginsbach C, Flechtenmacher C, Müller BT, Hort W, Stögbauer F, Hausser I: Ultrastrukturelle Untersuchungen in Arterien zur Pathogenese von Dissektionen. Akt Neurol 2000;27:S145(249).

16 Bacchelli B, Quaglino D, Gheduzzi D, Taparelli F, Boraldi F, Trolli B, Le Saux O, Boyd CD, Pasquali-Ronchetti I: Identification of heterozygote carriers in families with a recessive form of pseudoxanthoma elasticum (PXE). Mod Pathol 1999;12:1211–1223.

17 Grond-Ginsbach C, Schnippering H, Hausser I, Weber R, Werner I, Steiner H, Lüttgen N, Busse O, Grau A, Brandt T: Ultrastructural connective tissue aberrations in patients with intracranial aneurysms. Stroke 2002;33:2192–2196.
18 Hausser I, Grond-Ginsbach C, Orberk E, Tariverdian G, Brandt T: Nachweis ultrastruktureller Bindegewebsanomalien bei Familienangehörigen von Dissektionspatienten (abstract). Akt Neurol 1999;26:S103–S104.
19 Anderson RM, Schechter MM: A case of spontaneous dissecting aneurysm of the internal carotid artery. J Neurol Neurosurg Psychiatry 1959;22:195–201.
20 Thal DR, Schober R, Schlote W: Carotid artery dissection in a young adult: Cystic medial necrosis associated with an increased elastase content. Clin Neuropathol 1997;16:180–184.
21 Brandt T, Grond-Ginsbach C: Spontaneous cervical artery dissection – From risk factors towards pathogenesis (editorial). Stroke 2000;33:657–658.
22 Dunac A, Blecic S, Jeangette S, Bier JC, Rosetti P, Hildebrand JG: Stroke due to artery dissection: Role of collagen disease (abstract). Cerebrovasc Dis 1998;8(suppl 4):18.
23 Ulbricht D, Diederich J, Hermann-Le T, Metz RJ, Macian F, Pierard GE: Cervical artery dissection. An atypical presentation with Ehlers-Danlos like collagen pathology? Neurology 2004;63:1708–1710.

Priv.-Doz. Dr. med. Tobias Brandt, Med. Direktor
Neurologisches Fach- und Rehabilitationskrankenhaus Speyererhof
Kliniken Schmieder, DE–69117 Heidelberg (Germany)
Tel. +49 6221 6540 221, Fax +49 6221 6540 560
E-Mail T.Brandt@kliniken-schmieder.de

Baumgartner RW, Bogousslavsky J, Caso V, Paciaroni M (eds): Handbook on Cerebral Artery Dissection. Front Neurol Neurosci. Basel, Karger, 2005, vol 20, pp 30–43

Genetic Approaches in the Study of Risk Factors for Cervical Artery Dissection

Caspar Grond-Ginsbach[a], *Stéphanie Debette*[b], *Alessandro Pezzini*[c]

[a]Neurologische Klinik der Universität Heidelberg, Heidelberg, Deutschland;
[b]Clinique Neurologique, Hôpital Roger Salengro – CHRU, Lille, France;
[c]Clinica Neurologica, Università degli Studi di Brescia, Brescia, Italia

Abstract

The familial risk of spontaneous cervical artery dissections (sCAD) and the prevalence of the disease in the general population are not well known, making it difficult to estimate the importance of genetic risk factors in sCAD. sCAD is associated in rare cases with inherited diseases such as Ehlers-Danlos syndrome or osteogenesis imperfecta. In most instances, however, sCAD occurs in the absence of known heritable diseases. Genetic risk factors might play a role in further associated conditions, like the ultrastructural connective tissue alterations that are found in skin biopsies of most patients. Systematic mutation search in genes known for their implication in connective tissue disorders has been disappointing apart from rare missense mutations in the genes encoding type V collagen that were found in a minority of patients with sCAD. Efforts are now focusing on genetic linkage studies scanning the whole genome for markers that cosegregate with the above-mentioned dermal connective tissue alterations. Concomitantly, genetic association studies tested the association between sCAD and candidate genes that were selected a priori on pathophysiological arguments, in particular genes playing a role in the extracellular matrix, endothelial function, or inflammatory processes. Most association studies reported until now were negative, apart from one showing an association with a polymorphism in the MTHFR gene and another with a polymorphism in the ICAM-1 gene. However, the results of the association studies published so far must be interpreted cautiously because of the small sample sizes.

Evidence of a Genetic Predisposition to Develop a Cervical Artery Dissection

If there are genetic variants that predispose to a disease, a positive family history of that disease should be a risk factor for the disease itself. Stated another way, the disease should cluster within pedigrees if genetic risk factors exist.

Family history studies of multifactorial diseases vary considerably in design and scope. Many studies rely on unconfirmed test person reports to determine the disease status of family members. A more valid approach to characterizing disease status among all living pedigree members is by direct questioning of all members rather than relying on test person reports alone. Studies that rely only on responses to self-administered questionnaires are limited because they exclude fatal cases, whereas studies that rely only on data from death certificates are limited because they exclude nonfatal cases. As to family history studies of stroke, many of them did not distinguish hemorrhagic from ischemic stroke, very few attempted to differentiate the pathogenic subtypes of ischemic stroke [1–4] and none considered spontaneous cervical artery dissections (sCAD) as a distinct entity. Although this undoubtedly compromises the investigators' ability to detect an inherited component of sCAD, the results of the reported analyses suggest that inherited factors are involved in the pathogenesis of noncardioembolic strokes and that such an effect is more pronounced in younger individuals.

Familial Occurrence of sCAD

Reports on familial cervical artery dissections (CAD) are rare. Table 1 summarizes data on 11 families with 23 affected first-degree relatives. Two of the families were affected with a known connective tissue disorder, the other 9 families were without symptoms of such diseases.

The data from table 1 suggest an intrafamilial concordance of the localization [internal carolid artery (ICA) or vertebral artery (VA)] and of the age at the first dissection. Moreover, familial dissections tend to occur earlier in life (mean age in this series: 38.7 years, compared to a mean age of 42–44 years in two community-based studies [5, 6]) with an increased risk of recurrencies or multivessel events (35 dissections in 23 patients [7]). These findings suggest that the familial occurrence of CAD was not a matter of mere coincidence. Patients are likely to share common risk factors. Mutations in genes involved in the biosynthesis of type I and type III collagens are probably responsible for the increased risk for sCAD in the two families with a clinical phenotype of a connective tissue disorder (Ehlers-Danlos syndrome and osteogenesis imperfecta) [12, 13]. No genetic risk factors have been identified in the other families yet.

There are no published estimates of the prevalence of sCAD. However, the prevalence of patients who suffered from a CAD at least once during life can be deduced from data on the annual incidence of the disease. The overall annual incidence in two independent community-based studies has been estimated at 2.6 and 2.9 cases/100,000 population for all age groups, with mean ages of

Table 1. Patients with sCAD and with first-degree relatives also affected with sCAD

Mother (35 years) with bilateral ICA dissections, followed by a renal artery dissection 8 years later; daughter (18 years) with a right ICA dissection, followed by a left ICA dissection 5 years later [7, 8]
Father (76 years) with a right ICA dissection; son (47 years) with bilateral ICA dissections [7, 8]
Sister (25 years) with a left VA dissection, followed by a right VA dissection 6 years later; brother (25 years) with an ICA dissection [7]
Father (55 years) with a right ICA dissection, daughter (31 years) with a left ICA dissection; second daughter (38 years) with a right ICA dissection [9]
Brother (29 years) with a left VA dissection; sister (28 years) with a left VA dissection, followed by a right VA dissection 3 weeks later [10]
Father (31 years) with a left ICA dissection; son (30 years) with a left VA dissection, followed by a right VA dissection after one year, a right ICA dissection after 2 years, and a left ICA dissection after 3 years [10]
Brother (49 years) with a left ICA dissection; sister (59 years) with a left ICA dissection [11]
Sister (36 years) with a right VA dissection, followed by a left ICA dissection; sister (38 years) with a right VA dissection [10]
Father (53 years) with a left VA dissection; daughter (29 years) with a right ICA dissection [10]
Brother (47 years) with a right ICA dissection, followed by a left ICA dissection 7 years later; sister (42 years) with a left ICA dissection (family with clinical diagnosis of osteogenesis imperfecta) [12]
Daughter (34 years) with bilateral ICA and VA dissections; mother (45 years) with ICA dissection (family with clinical diagnosis of Ehlers-Danlos syndrome type IV) [13]

44 and 42 years, respectively [5, 6]. Assuming a (hardly decreased) life expectancy of 30 years after the dissection, the prevalence of sCAD survivors is about 0.8/1,000. Under these assumptions, the probability for an index patient to have at least one affected first-degree relative (under the assumption of a mean-sized family of 2 parents, 2 sibs and 2 children) as a pure coincidence is about $1 - (1 - 0.0008)^6 = 1 - 0.9992^6 =$ about 4.8/1,000 or roughly one in 200.

Epidemiological data on the familial occurrence of sCAD are scarce. No patients with a familial history of CAD were found in a series of 352 patients from Zürich-Bern [14] (Baumgartner, pers. commun.). In the Basel CAD registry one pair of siblings was recorded among 98 CAD patients (Engelter, pers. commun.). Schievink et al. [7] included three pairs of familial cases in their review of medical records from 175 patients. These sparse data do not enable a proper estimation of the prevalence of familial cases. It is even less possible to compare the observed prevalence with the expected prevalence on the basis of mere coincidence and estimate the overall contribution of genetic factors to the development of sCAD.

Association of sCAD with Hereditary Connective Tissue Syndromes (Marfan Syndrome, Ehlers-Danlos Syndrome, Osteogenesis imperfecta, Pseudoxanthoma elasticum)

In a French multicenter study 3 out of 459 patients were found to have a documented Marfan syndrome. No patients with other inherited connective tissue disorders were reported [15]. In a consecutive series of 276 Swiss patients with CAD, Marfan syndrome was observed in a single patient and no clinical evidence of Ehlers-Danlos syndrome type IV, pseudoxanthoma elasticum, osteogenesis imperfecta or polycystic kidney disease was found [14]. Thus, patients with known hereditary connective tissue disorders are apparently rare amongst patients with sCAD. However, sCAD might be associated with unknown (subtypes of known) connective tissue disorders. Indeed, Schievink et al. [16] described 3 patients with subtle heritable connective tissue signs in a small prospective study of 15 patients with sCAD and dermal connective tissue alterations were described in most patients with sCAD [17–20]. Mayer et al. [21] described a patient with a COL1A1 mutation and spontaneous multivessel CAD and with clinical signs of mild osteogenesis imperfecta.

The contribution of genetic factors is probably not equally important in all patients. In a minority of patients we may find known or unknown Mendelian disorders (such as in the families with osteogenesis imperfecta or Ehlers-Danlos syndrome type IV or with clinical symptoms of other connective tissue disorders). In the majority of patients we might perhaps detect genetic polymorphisms with a minor effect on the development of sCAD. The identification and the analysis of such genetic variants require high methodological and technical standards. It is not unlikely that a further clinical differentiation of the patients into more homogeneous phenotypes will enhance the power of subsequent genetic studies: exclusion of traumatic dissections, differentiation between VA dissections and ICA dissections, between patients with or without minor signs of a connective tissue disorder, etc.

Mutation Search in Patients with sCAD

Candidate genes for mutation search in patients with CAD were mainly selected on the basis of a presumed association between CAD and known connective tissue disorders and of the finding of connective tissue abnormalities in skin biopsies of patients. Genes known to carry the mutations responsible for vascular and classical Ehlers-Danlos syndrome and for pseudoxanthoma elasticum were analyzed in patients with sCAD, as well as further genes involved in the biosynthesis or the remodeling of extracellular matrix components.

Table 2. Mutation search in patients with a cervical artery dissection

Gene	Patients, n	Result	References
ABCC6	12	no mutation	[22]
COL3A1	18	no mutation	[23]
COL3A1	12	no mutation	[9]
COL5A1	19	D192N in one patient	[24]
COL5A2	10	1× T1227S/1× D1429V 1× V509A + P830L	[25]
COL8A1	13	no mutation	[26]
COL8A2	13	no mutation	[26]
ELN	10	no mutation	[27]

No relevant mutations were found in COL8A1, COL8A2, DCN, ELN, and ABCC6 (table 2). The significance of the missense mutations found in COL5A1 and COL5A2 is unclear. Exon skip mutations and mutations in the COL5A1 and COL5A2 genes that encode glycine substitutions were found in patients with the classical type of Ehlers-Danlos syndrome. It is conceivable that other variants in these genes increase the risk for dissections and it was recently proposed that patients with sCAD suffer from an unknown and mild type of Ehlers-Danlos syndrome [19]. However, whether the missense mutations in COL5A1 or COL5A2 that were found in some patients with sCAD are disease causing or just genetic variants with or without disease-modifying effect is a matter of pure speculation.

The number of patients analyzed in mutation screens was necessarily small. The value of the mutation search studies, therefore, strongly depends on the selection of representative patients. These studies indicate, that variants in the analyzed genes are not common amongst sCAD patients, but they do not rule out that mutations in these genes play a decisive role in a minority of the patients or in an etiological subgroup such as cases with VA dissection, or patients with multiple dissection, or with accompanying signs of connective tissue alterations.

Genetic Association Studies

Association studies test the association between a disease and a genetic polymorphism. They usually do not require family data. In brief they test for significant differences in allele and genotype frequencies between affected individuals and control subjects. The power to detect a genetic association depends on the number of subjects, the strength of the association, and the frequency of the studied polymorphism. Control subjects and patients must be sampled from the same ethnic population. Indeed, comparing patients and controls with different ethnic origins can lead to spurious associations, that is to the detection of an association that does not exist. Finally, studies that detect a significant association between a phenotype and a genetic polymorphism in a certain population should be reproduced and confirmed in independent samples from other populations [28, 29].

In complex and probably multifactorial diseases like sCAD, several polymorphisms each with a small size effect rather than one major gene with a strong effect are to be expected. Most studies published until now failed to detect associations and the few associations that have been found could not be reproduced in other studies. However, these studies obviously lacked statistical power and were all based on relatively small samples. The detection of realistic odd ratios of 1.2–1.5 with a statistical power of 80% requires at least several hundreds of subjects in each group. Moreover, multifactorial diseases also have environmental risk factors that can interact with the genetic predisposing factors. This makes the detection of genetic predisposing factors even more difficult, especially if the environmental risk factors cannot be taken into account in the statistical analysis (because they were not determined or because they are unknown).

Several research groups have tested a possible association between the MTHFR 677TT genotype and sCAD (table 3). Mildly increased plasma levels of homocysteine are found in patients with sCAD. Hyperhomocysteinemia was considered as a potential risk factor for CAD following chiropractic manipulation of the cervical spine [41]. Interestingly, elevated plasma homocysteine levels are also associated with endothelial dysfunction and cardiovascular diseases. The homozygous TT genotype of the T677C polymorphism in the MTHFR gene (encoding the thermolabile form of the enzyme) is associated with mild hyperhomocysteinemia. A significant association of sCAD with the 677TT genotype was found in a small prospective Italian case control study [32], whereas another Italian study reported a nonsignificant trend towards a preponderance of the T allele amongst a series of consecutive patients [38]. However, this trend was not confirmed in two subsequent German studies with more patients but with less stringent designs [33, 39]. The relationship of sCAD with decreased α-1-antitrypsin levels was studied by several authors [11, 30, 42–44], but the results are not yet definite.

Some further genes (Toll-like receptor 4, coagulation factors II, V, and VII, CD40, CD154) were analyzed in association studies with young stroke patients including a subgroup of patients with sCAD [45–47]. Most promising are the results by Longoni et al. [34] in a series of 96 patients with CAD. The observed association of sCAD with the GG genotype of the A469G polymorphism of the

Table 3. Genetic association studies in patients with sCAD and matched healthy control subjects

Gene	Patients, n	Controls, n	Result	References
AAT (PiZ,PiS)	74	74	no significant association	[11]
AAT (PiZ,PiS)	80	80	no significant association	[30]
ApoE ($\varepsilon2$ $\varepsilon3$ $\varepsilon4$)	11	16	no significant association	[31]
CBS (844 ins)	25	36	no significant association	[32]
CBS (844 ins)	95	95	no significant association	[33]
COL3A1	45	50	no significant association	[9]
ICAM-1 (469)	96	204	association ($p < 0.01$)	[34]
IL6 (promoter)	56	56	no significant association	[35]
IL8 (promoter)	20	21	no significant association	[36]
MMP9 (promoter)	52	52	no significant association	[37]
MTHFD1 (1958)	95	95	no significant association	[33]
MTHFR (677)	26	30	no significant association	[38]
MTHFR (677)	25	36	association ($p < 0.05$)	[32]
MTHFR (677)	94	30	no significant association	[39]
MTHFR (677)	95	95	no significant association	[33]
Prot Z (promoter)	37	199	no significant association	[40]

ICAM-1 gene (CD54) suggests a role for initial processes of inflammation. This finding is in line with earlier studies showing an association of sCAD with infections [42, 48]. Indeed, infections are frequently reported during the weeks preceding the dissection and are considered as an independent risk factor. Hence, genetic variants that are known to modulate the infection susceptibility as well as the inflammatory response are interesting candidates. Also the finding of significantly higher C-reactive protein levels in a small series of sCAD survivors compared to other stroke survivors indicates a role of proinflammatory processes in the pathogenesis of sCAD [49, 50].

Several researchers observed an association between a history of migraine and sCAD [51–53]. Given the strong influence of genetic factors in the development of migraine one can speculate that these two disorders might share some susceptibility genes and that progress made in the genetic analysis of migraine might stimulate the genetic analysis of sCAD. An association between sCAD and intracranial aneurysms was reported [54, 55] and similar ultrastructural connective tissue alterations were also found in skin biopsies from patients with intracranial aneurysms [56]. Amongst the different loci that were recently proposed for intracranial aneurysms [57–59], there might be candidate loci for sCAD, too. However, the association of intracranial aneurysms and sCAD was not confirmed in 162 sCAD patients from Zürich-Bern, who underwent cerebral catheter angiography, magnetic resonance angiography, or both [14].

Intermediate Phenotypes in Patients with sCAD

The dissecting event in the arterial wall is thought to precede the subsequent clinical signs for hours or even days. The origin of the intramural blood is unknown in most cases [60]. (However, autopsy findings and a review of the literature suggest that an intimal tear is the most likely cause of the intramural hematoma [Baumgartner, pers. commun.].) It is not clear whether a dissection develops abruptly into a normal healthy arterial wall (for instance, due to mechanical trauma), or whether long lasting pathological processes have changed the structure of the arterial wall and increased the risk for vascular tears. Moreover, we do not know whether most dissections have a common etiology, or whether different subtypes must be individualized. The concordance of the few familial cases of dissection suggests that VA and ICA have specific pathogenetic factors. Intermediate phenotypes might be valuable for the genetic analysis of sCAD as a complex clinical disorder with assumed genetic heterogeneity [20, 61, 62]. An intermediate phenotype is a condition that predisposes to sCAD and can be subclinical (e.g. reduced type III collagen synthesis in fibroblasts, morphological alteration in the dermal connective tissue, impaired endothelial function, increased arterial stiffness). Intermediate phenotypes are particularly valuable when they are easy to measure, quantifiable, less heterogeneous than sCAD, and not too rare. This increases the chances of detecting genetic predisposing factors. Some intermediate phenotypes may have a Mendelian inheritance, thus permitting classical genetic linkage analysis. The two following intermediate phenotypes were used for genetic studies during the last years.

Type III Collagen Synthesis in Fibroblasts

A reduced production of type III collagen may predispose to the formation of sCAD in some patients [63]. A reduction of type III collagen synthesis was also found in fibroblasts from patients with intracranial aneurysms. However, mutations in COL3A1, the gene that encodes type III collagen, were not found. van den Berg et al. [64] analyzed a family with intracranial aneurysms and found reduced synthesis of type III collagen in the affected members. Genetic linkage analysis with a polymorph genetic marker excluded the COL3A1 locus as possible mutation locus for this family with intracranial aneurysms. This intermediate phenotype was not yet analyzed in a kindred with familial dissections.

Morphological Alterations in the Dermal Connective Tissue

Many patients with sCAD have morphological alterations in their dermal connective tissue that resemble the findings in patients with Ehlers-Danlos syndrome or in heterozygous carriers of pseudoxanthoma elasticum [20]. Some kindreds with an autosomal dominant inheritance of the dermal connective tissue phenotype were described. Perhaps part of the patients with sCAD might be affected with mild subtypes of known connective tissue disorders [19, 20, 65].

Exclusion mapping in a small family ruled out most candidate genes that were proposed on the basis of pathophysiological assumptions [66]. Suggestive linkage in chromosome region 15q2 was found in a genome-wide scan of one family with inherited dermal connective tissue alterations. This latter candidate region contains several interesting candidate genes [67]. The region is composed of several long repeated sequences, that contain multiple copies of parts of neighbored gene families (pseudogenes of GLP, GCSP4, Dynamin) [68] which makes mutation search particularly difficult, as the specific amplification of highly homologous sequence copies is technically hard. Interestingly, a duplication of this chromosome region was recently found in patients with panic disorders and hypermobility [69]. However, the presence of this duplication was not confirmed by others and might be a technical artifact, caused by the presence of multiple repeat sequences within this region [70–72].

Further subclinical phenotypes were shown to be associated with sCAD, such as impaired endothelial function [73], increased arterial stiffness [74], and aortic root dilation [75, 76]. They have not been used yet as intermediate phenotypes for genetic studies of sCAD.

Discussion

Although the existence of a genetic predisposition to sCAD is not convincingly proven, the number of molecular and genetic studies of this disease increases rapidly. Despite the fact that these studies have not yet been able to consistently find a genetic predisposing factor to sCAD, they have certainly improved our understanding of the disease. The demonstration of an association of sCAD with previous infections and with migraine will stimulate further genetic analysis. The association with dermal connective tissue alterations inherited with an autosomal dominant pattern is among the most promising results. Furthermore, even though they could not yet be replicated, the associations described with polymorphisms in the MTHFR and the ICAM-1 gene deserve close attention.

Insufficient sample sizes is the most important shortcoming of genetic studies on sCAD, mostly due to the low incidence rates of the disease. Indeed, sCAD is probably a multifactorial disease with several genetic predisposing factors each having a small size effect rather than one major gene with a strong effect. To increase their statistical power, future genetic association studies should thus aim at larger sample sizes, possibly through multicenter collaborations. Besides, the phenotype of the patients included in these studies should be thoroughly described and the control subjects carefully matched. Differentiating between different clinical subtypes and taking into account environmental risk factors might as well prove useful.

Future research should also focus on intermediate phenotypes, such as the dermal connective tissue phenotype, which is associated with sCAD and segregates with an autosomal dominant pattern. Indeed, the Mendelian inheritance pattern is an ideal setting for linkage studies that scan the whole genome for loci that cosegregate with the disease, without any a priori hypothesis on the underlying pathophysiology. Here again, the power to detect a linkage increases with the number of families studied.

Finally, a systematic assessment of the familial risk of sCAD (that has never been performed until now) would help us estimate more precisely the contribution of genetic risk factors to this complex disease.

Acknowledgments

We thank Drs. Marie-Luise Arnold, Tobias Brandt, Stefan Engelter, Werner Hacke, Ingrid Hausser, Christoph Lichy, and Philippe Lyrer for critical reading of the manuscript. Drs. Ralf Baumgartner and Stefan Engelter are acknowledged for information on the occurrence of familial dissections among their patients.

References

1 Meschia JF, Brown RD Jr, Brott TG, Hardy J, Atkinson EJ, O'Brien PC: Feasibility of an affected sibling pair study in ischemic stroke: Results of a 2-center family history registry. Stroke 2001;32:2939–2941.

2 Polychronopoulos P, Gioldasis G, Ellul J, Metallinos IC, Lekka NP, Paschalis C, Papapetropoulos T: Family history of stroke in stroke types and subtypes. J Neurol Sci 2002;195:117–122.

3 Schulz UG, Flossmann E, Rothwell PM: Heritability of ischemic stroke in relation to age, vascular risk factors, and subtypes of incident stroke in population-based studies. Stroke 2004;35: 819–824.

4 Flossmann E, Schulz UG, Rothwell PM: Systematic review of methods and results of studies of the genetic epidemiology of ischemic stroke. Stroke 2004;35:212–227.

5 Schievink WI, Mokri B, Whisnant JP: Internal carotid artery dissection in a community. Rochester, Minnesota, 1987–1992. Stroke 1993;24:1678–1680.

6 Giroud M, Fayolle H, Andre N, Dumas R, Becker F, Martin D, Baudoin N, Krause D: Incidence of internal carotid artery dissection in the community of Dijon. J Neurol Neurosurg Psychiatry 1994; 57:1443.

7 Schievink WI, Mokri B, Piepgras DG, Kuiper JD: Recurrent spontaneous arterial dissections: Risk in familial versus nonfamilial disease. Stroke 1996;27:622–624.
8 Mokri B, Piepgras DG, Wiebers DO, Houser OW: Familial occurrence of spontaneous dissection of the internal carotid artery. Stroke 1987;18:246–251.
9 von Pein F, Valkkila M, Schwarz R, Morcher M, Klima B, Grau A, Ala-Kokko L, Hausser I, Brandt T, Grond-Ginsbach C: Analysis of the COL3A1 gene in patients with spontaneous cervical artery dissections. J Neurol 2002;249:862–866.
10 Martin JJ, Hausser I, Weber R, Engelter S, Lyrer P, Busse O, Schwarz R, Brandt T, Hacke W, Grond-Ginsbach C: Familial cervical artery dissections – Clinical and genetical investigations. Cerebrovasc Dis 2004;17(suppl 5):72.
11 Grond-Ginsbach C, Engelter S, Werner I, Hausser I, Müller U, Brandt T, Lyrer P: Alpha-1-antitrypsin deficiency alleles are not associated with cervical artery dissections. Neurology 2004;62: 1190–1192.
12 Rouviere S, Michelini R, Sarda P, Pages M: Spontaneous carotid artery dissection in two siblings with osteogenesis imperfecta. Cerebrovasc Dis 2004;17:270–272.
13 Mondon K, de Toffol B, Georgesco G, Cassarini JF, Machet MC, Cottier JP, Arbeille B, Autret A: Dissection simultanées des deux artères carotides internes et des deux artères vertébrales révélatrices d'un Syndrome d'Ehlers-Danlos type IV. Rev Neurol (Paris) 2004;160:478–482.
14 Benninger D, Georgiadis D, Arnold M, Baumgartner RW: Prevalence of hereditary connective tissue disorders, intracranial aneurysms and fibromuscular dysplasia in spontaneous carotid artery dissection. Cerebrovasc Dis 2004;17(suppl 5):92.
15 Touze E, Gauvrit JY, Moulin T, Meder JF, Bracard S, Mas JL; multicenter survey on natural history of cervical artery dissection: Risk of stroke and recurrent dissection after a cervical artery dissection: A multicenter study. Neurology 2003;61:1347–1351.
16 Schievink WI, Wijdicks EF, Michels VV, Vockley J, Godfrey M: Heritable connective tissue disorders in cervical artery dissections: A prospective study. Neurology 1998;50:1166–1169.
17 Brandt T, Hausser I, Orberk E, Grau A, Hartschuh W, Anton-Lamprecht I, Hacke W: Ultrastructural connective tissue abnormalities in patients with spontaneous cervicocerebral artery dissections. Ann Neurol 1998;44:281–285.
18 Brandt T, Orberk E, Weber R, Werner I, Busse O, Muller B, Wigger F, Grau A, Grond-Ginsbach C, Hausser I: Pathogenesis of cervical artery dissections: Association with connective tissue abnormalities. Neurology 2001;57:24–30.
19 Ulbricht D, Diederich NJ, Hermanns-Le T, Metz RJ, Macian F, Pierard GE: Cervical artery dissection: An atypical presentation with Ehlers-Danlos-like collagen pathology? Neurology 2004;63: 1708–1710.
20 Hausser I, Muller U, Engelter S, Lyrer P, Pezzini A, Padovani A, Moormann B, Busse O, Weber R, Brandt T, Grond-Ginsbach C: Different types of connective tissue alterations associated with cervical artery dissections. Acta Neuropathol (Berl) 2004;107:509–514.
21 Mayer SA, Rubin BS, Starman BJ, Byers PH: Spontaneous multivessel cervical artery dissection in a patient with a substitution of alanine for glycine (G13A) in the alpha 1 (I) chain of type I collagen. Neurology 1996;47:552–526.
22 Morcher M, Hausser I, Brandt T, Grond-Ginsbach C: Heterozygous carriers of pseudoxanthoma elasticum were not found among patients with cervical artery dissections. J Neurol 2003;250: 983–986.
23 Kuivaniemi H, Prockop DJ, Wu Y, Madhatheri SL, Kleinert C, Earley JJ, Jokinen A, Stolle C, Majamaa K, Myllyla VV, et al: Exclusion of mutations in the gene for type III collagen (COL3A1) as a common cause of intracranial aneurysms or cervical artery dissections: Results from sequence analysis of the coding sequences of type III collagen from 55 unrelated patients. Neurology 1993;43:2652–2658.
24 Grond-Ginsbach C, Weber R, Haas J, Orberk E, Kunz S, Busse O, Hausser I, Brandt T, Wildemann B: Mutations in the COL5A1 coding sequence are not common in patients with spontaneous cervical artery dissections. Stroke 1999;30:1887–1890.
25 Grond-Ginsbach C, Wigger F, Morcher M, von Pein F, Grau A, Hausser I, Brandt T: Sequence analysis of the COL5A2 gene in patients with spontaneous cervical artery dissections. Neurology 2002;58:1103–1105.

26 Kuhlenbaumer G, Muller US, Besselmann M, Rauterberg J, Robenek H, Hunermund G, Brandt T, Ringelstein EB, Stogbauer F, Hausser I: Neither collagen 8A1 nor 8A2 mutations play a major role in cervical artery dissection. A mutation analysis and linkage study. J Neurol 2004;251:357–359.
27 Grond-Ginsbach C, Thomas-Feles C, Werner I, Weber R, Wigger F, Hausser I, Brandt T: Mutations in the tropoelastin gene (ELN) were not found in patients with spontaneous cervical artery dissections. Stroke 2000;31:1935–1938.
28 Ioannidis JP: Genetic associations: False or true? Trends Mol Med 2003;9:135–138.
29 Ioannidis JP, Trikalinos TA, Ntzani EE, Contopoulos-Ioannidis DG: Genetic associations in large versus small studies: An empirical assessment. Lancet 2003;361:567–571.
30 Konrad C, Langer C, Muller GA, Berger K, Dziewas R, Stogbauer F, Nabavi DG, Junker R, Ringelstein EB, Kuhlenbaumer G: Protease inhibitors in spontaneous cervical artery dissections. Stroke 2005;36: in press.
31 Orlandi G, Fanucchi S, Mancuso M, Gelli A, Rocchi A, Siciliano G, Murri L: Dissection and atherosclerosis of carotid arteries in the young: Role of the apolipoprotein E polymorphism. Eur J Neurol 2002;9:19–21.
32 Pezzini A, Del Zotto E, Archetti S, Negrini R, Bani P, Albertini A, Grassi M, Assanelli D, Gasparotti R, Vignolo LA, Magoni M, Padovani A: Plasma homocysteine concentration, C677T MTHFR genotype, and 844ins68bp CBS genotype in young adults with spontaneous cervical artery dissection and atherothrombotic stroke. Stroke 2002;33:664–669.
33 Konrad C, Muller GA, Langer C, Kuhlenbaumer G, Berger K, Nabavi DG, Dziewas R, Stogbauer F, Ringelstein EB, Junker R: Plasma homocysteine, MTHFR C677T, CBS 844ins68bp, and MTHFD1 G1958A polymorphisms in spontaneous cervical artery dissections. J Neurol 2004;251: 1242–1248.
34 Longoni M, Lichy C, Schwaninger M, Ferrarese C, Grond-Ginsbach C: ICAM-1 A469G polymorphism is a risk factor for juvenile cerebral ischemia due to arterial dissection. Eur J Neurol 2004;11(suppl 2):52.
35 Wiest T, Werner I, Brandt T, Grond-Ginsbach C: Interleukin 6 (IL6) promoter variants in patients with spontaneous cervical artery dissections. Cerebrovasc Dis 2004;17:347–348.
36 Grau AJ, Aulmann M, Lichy C, Meiser H, Buggle F, Brandt T, Grond-Ginsbach C: Increased cytokine release by leucocytes in survivors of stroke at young age. Eur J Clin Invest 2001;31: 999–1006.
37 Wagner S, Kluge B, Koziol J, Grau A, Grond-Ginsbach C: MMP-9 polymorphisms are not associated with spontaneous cervical artery dissection. Stroke 2004;35:e62–e64.
38 Gallai V, Caso V, Paciaroni M, Cardaioli G, Arning E, Bottiglieri T, Parnetti L: Mild hyperhomocyst(e)inemia: A possible risk factor for cervical artery dissection. Stroke 2001;32:714–718.
39 Mueller U, Wiest T, Grau A, Brandt T, Grond-Ginsbach C: Gene polymorphisms causing mild hyperhomocysteinaemia and thrombophilia – Possible risk factors for spontaneous cervical artery dissections. Cerebrovasc Dis 2003;16(suppl 4):75.
40 Lichy C, Kropp S, Dong-Si T, Genius J, Dolan T, Hampe T, Stoll F, Reuner K, Grond-Ginsbach C, Grau A: A common polymorphism of the protein Z gene is associated with protein Z plasma levels and with risk of cerebral ischemia in the young. Stroke 2004;35:40–45.
41 Pezzini A, Del Zotto E, Padovani A: Hyperhomocysteinemia: A potential risk factor for cervical artery dissection following chiropractic manipulation of the cervical spine. J Neurol 2002;249: 1401–1403.
42 Grau AJ, Brandt T, Buggle F, Orberk E, Mytilineos J, Werle E, Conradt, Krause M, Winter R, Hacke W: Association of cervical artery dissection with recent infection. Arch Neurol 1999;56: 851–856.
43 Pezzini A, Magoni M, Corda L, Pini L, Medicina D, Crispino M, Pavia M, Padovani A, Grassi V: Alpha-1-antitrypsin-deficiency-associated cervical artery dissection: Report of three cases. Eur Neurol 2002;47:201–204.
44 Vila N, Millan M, Ferrer X, Riutort N, Escudero D: Levels of alpha1-antitrypsin in plasma and risk of spontaneous cervical artery dissections: A case-control study. Stroke 2003;34:E168–E169.
45 Reismann P, Lichy C, Rudofsky G, Humpert PM, Genius J, Si TD, Dorfer C, Grau AJ, Hamann A, Hacke W, Nawroth PP, Bierhaus A: Lack of association between polymorphisms of the toll-like receptor 4 gene and cerebral ischemia. J Neurol 2004;251:853–858.

46 Lichy C, Stoll F, Kropp S, Genius J, Dong-Si T, Reuner K, Litfin F, Grau A: Cerebral ischemia in young adults and genetic polymorphisms of coagulation factors II, V and VII. Thromb Haemost 2004;91:825–827.

47 Debette S, Lichy C, Genius J, Dong-Si T, Stoll F, Werner I, Grau AJ, Leys D, Hacke W, Grond-Ginsbach C: CD40/CD40L genetic variants and cerebral ischemia of the young. Cerebrovasc Dis 2004;17(suppl 5):85.

48 Guillon B, Berthet K, Benslamia L, Bertrand M, Bousser MG, Tzourio C: Infection and the risk of spontaneous cervical artery dissection: A case-control study. Stroke 2003;34:e79–e81.

49 Genius J, Grau AJ, Lichy C: CRP levels are elevated in cerebral ischemia due to cervical arterial dissection. Cerebrovasc Dis 2004;17(suppl 5):11.

50 Genius J, Dong-Si T, Grau AJ, Lichy C: Postacute CRP levels are elevated in cervical artery dissection. Stroke 2005;in press.

51 Tzourio C, Benslamia L, Guillon B, Aidi S, Bertrand M, Berthet K, Bousser MG: Migraine and the risk of cervical artery dissection: A case-control study. Neurology 2002;59:435–437.

52 Granella F, Pezzini A, Zanferrari C, Del Zotto E, Bertolino C, Bazzoli E: Migraine without aura is a major risk factor for cervical artery dissection. A case-control study. Cephalalgia 2003;23:571.

53 Pezzini A, Granella F, Grassi M, Bertolino C, Del Zotto E, Immovilli P, Bazzoli E, Padovani A, Zanferrari C: History of migraine and the risk of spontaneous cervical artery dissection. Cephalalgia 2005;in press.

54 Schievink WI, Mokri B, Michels VV, Piepgras DG: Familial association of intracranial aneurysms and cervical artery dissections. Stroke 1991;22:1426–1430.

55 Majamaa K, Portimojarvi H, Sotaniemi KA, Myllyla VV: Familial aggregation of cervical artery dissection and cerebral aneurysm. Stroke 1994;25:1704–1705.

56 Grond-Ginsbach C, Schnippering H, Hausser I, Weber R, Werner I, Steiner HH, Luttgen N, Busse O, Grau A, Brandt T: Ultrastructural connective tissue aberrations in patients with intracranial aneurysms. Stroke 2002;33:2192–2196.

57 Roos YB, Pals G, Struycken PM, Rinkel GJ, Limburg M, Pronk JC, van den Berg JS, Luijten JA, Pearson PL, Vermeulen M, Westerveld A: Genome-wide linkage in a large Dutch consanguineous family maps a locus for intracranial aneurysms to chromosome 2p13. Stroke 2004;35:2276–22781.

58 van der Voet M, Olson JM, Kuivaniemi H, Dudek DM, Skunca M, Ronkainen A, Niemela M, Jaaskelainen J, Hernesniemi J, Helin K, Leinonen E, Biswas M, Tromp G: Intracranial aneurysms in Finnish families: Confirmation of linkage and refinement of the interval to chromosome 19q13.3. Am J Hum Genet 2004;74:564–571.

59 Nahed BV, Seker A, Guclu B, Ozturk AK, Finberg K, Hawkins AA, Diluna ML, State M, Lifton RP, Gunel M: Mapping a Mendelian form of intracranial aneurysm to 1p34.3-p36.13. Am J Hum Genet 2005;76:172–179.

60 Schievink W: Spontaneous dissection of the carotid and vertebral arteries. N Engl J Med 2001; 344:898–906.

61 Brandt T, Grond-Ginsbach C: Spontaneous cervical artery dissection – From risk factors towards pathogenesis. Stroke 2002;33:657–658.

62 Pezzini A, Hausser I, Brandt T, Padovani A, Grond-Ginsbach C: Internal carotid artery dissection after French horn playing. Spontaneous or traumatic event? J Neurol 2003;250:1004–1005.

63 van den Berg JS, Limburg M, Kappelle LJ, Pals G, Arwert F, Westerveld A: The role of type III collagen in spontaneous cervical arterial dissections. Ann Neurol 1998;43:494–498.

64 van den Berg JS, Limburg M, Pals G, Arwert F, Westerveld A. Type III collagen deficiency in a family with intracranial aneurysms. Cerebrovasc Dis 2001;11:92–94.

65 Ogura K, Maegaki Y, Morino S, Ogawa T, Ohno K, Oka A: Vertebral artery dissection in an infant: Ultrastructural aberrations in connective tissue components. Neuropediatrics 2003;34:307–310.

66 Grond-Ginsbach C, Klima B, Weber R, Striegel J, Fischer C, Hacke W, Brandt T, Hausser I: Exclusion mapping of the genetic predisposition for cervical artery dissections by linkage analysis. Ann Neurol 2002;52:359–364.

67 Hyrenbach S, Bambul P, Wiest T, Moormann B, Pezzini A, Busse O, Hausser I, Brandt T, Grond-Ginsbach C: Suggestive linkage of a putative genetic risk factor for cervical artery dissections to chromosome region 15q2. Akt Neurol 2004;31(suppl 1):P526.

68 Pujana MA, Nadal M, Gratacos M, Peral B, Csiszar K, Gonzalez-Sarmiento R, Sumoy L, Estivill X: Additional complexity on human chromosome 15q: Identification of a set of newly recognized duplicons (LCR15) on 15q11-q13, 15q24, and 15q26. Genome Res 2001;11:98–111.

69 Gratacos M, Nadal M, Martin-Santos R, Pujana MA, Gago J, Peral B, Armengol L, Ponsa I, Miro R, Bulbena A, Estivill X: A polymorphic genomic duplication on human chromosome 15 is a susceptibility factor for panic and phobic disorders. Cell 2001;106:367–379.

70 Schumacher J, Otte AC, Becker T, Sun Y, Wienker TF, Wirth B, Franke P, Abou Jamra R, Propping P, Deckert J, Nothen MM, Cichon S: No evidence for DUP25 in patients with panic disorder using a quantitative real-time PCR approach. Hum Genet 2003;114:115–117.

71 Tabiner M, Youings S, Dennis N, Baldwin D, Buis C, Mayers A, Jacobs PA, Crolla JA: Failure to find DUP25 in patients with anxiety disorders, in control individuals, or in previously reported positive control cell lines. Am J Hum Genet 2003;72:535–538.

72 Vermeulen SJ, Menten B, De Bie S, Coucke P, Loeys B, Malfait F, De Backer J, Speleman F, De Paepe A: DUP25 remains unconfirmed. Am J Med Genet 2004;131A:320–321.

73 Lucas C, Lecroart JL, Gautier C, Leclerc X, Dauzat M, Leys D, Deklunder G: Impairment of endothelial function in patients with spontaneous cervical artery dissection: Evidence for a general arterial wall disease. Cerebrovasc Dis 2004;17:170–174.

74 Calvet D, Boutouyrie P, Touze E, Laloux B, Mas JL, Laurent S: Increased stiffness of the carotid wall material in patients with spontaneous cervical artery dissection. Stroke 2004;35:2078–2082.

75 Tzourio C, Cohen A, Lamisse N, Biousse V, Bousser MG: Aortic root dilatation in patients with spontaneous cervical artery dissection. Circulation 1997;95:2351–2353.

76 Skljarevski V, Turek M, Hakin AM: Cervical artery dissection is associated with widened aortic root diameter. Can J Neurol Sci 1998;25:315–319.

Dr. Caspar Grond-Ginsbach
Department of Neurology, University of Heidelberg
Im Neuenheimer Feld 400
DE–69120 Heidelberg (Germany)
Tel. +49 6221 568213, Fax +49 6221 565461
E-Mail Caspar_Grond-Ginsbach@med.uni-heidelberg.de

Baumgartner RW, Bogousslavsky J, Caso V, Paciaroni M (eds): Handbook on Cerebral Artery Dissection. Front Neurol Neurosci. Basel, Karger, 2005, vol 20, pp 44–53

Environmental Factors and Cervical Artery Dissection

Valeria Caso[a], *Maurizio Paciaroni*[a], *Julien Bogousslavsky*[b]

[a]Stroke Unit, Division of Internal and Cardiovascular Medicine, University of Perugia, Perugia, Italy; [b]Department of Neurology, Centre Hospitalier Universitaire Vaudois, Lausanne, Switzerland

Abstract

A history of a minor precipitating event is frequently elicited in patients with a spontaneous dissection of the carotid or vertebral artery. Other precipitating events associated with hyperextension or rotation of the neck include practicing yoga, painting a ceiling, coughing, vomiting, sneezing, the receipt of anesthesia, and the act of resuscitation. Chiropractic manipulation of the neck has been associated with carotid artery dissection and, particularly, vertebral artery dissection. Another risk factor for spontaneous dissections seems to be a recent history of a respiratory tract infection. The possibility of an infectious trigger is supported by the finding of a seasonal variation in the incidence of spontaneous dissections, with a peak incidence in fall. A potential link with common risk factors for vascular disease, such as tobacco use, hypertension, and the use of oral contraceptives, has not been systematically evaluated, but atherosclerosis appears to be distinctly uncommon in patients with a dissection of the carotid or vertebral arteries. In conclusion, although any hypotheses on the pathogenic mechanisms linking environmental factors and dissection remain speculative at present, we believe that these hypotheses may contribute to better define the spectrum of pathogenic conditions predisposing a cervical artery to dissection and provide arguments to better investigate the single or combined effect of such susceptibility factors in future studies.

Currently, the etiology of spontaneous cervical artery dissection (sCAD) is poorly understood. The genetic diseases responsible for sCAD are discussed in the chapters by Brandt et al. (pp. 16–29) and Grond-Ginsbach et al. (pp. 30–43), and traumatic CAD in the chapter by Nedeltchev and Baumgartner (pp. 71–77). When all known genetic diseases associated with dissection have been excluded and a major trauma did not occur, sCAD is often labeled as 'spontaneous' or 'idiopathic'. However, different precipitating events have been described as so-called minor traumas, which are believed to lead to sCAD [1]. According to Norris and Beletsky [2], the relationship between minor trauma and sCAD mainly depends on how well the patient's history is elicited. Although it is sometimes arbitrary to distinguish between major and minor trauma, it is assumed that events, which are usually not followed by sCAD (e.g. sneezing, coughing, vomiting, sport, and recreational activities) are minor trauma. Iatrogenic sCAD is also assumed to result from minor trauma, as dissection is a rare complication of diagnostic and therapeutic interventions. Other environmental risk factors for sCAD are recent infection and migraine, whereas the role of the season and vascular risk factors is less clear.

The aim of this chapter is to discuss most 'conventional' environmental risk factors for sCAD, including activities associated with sCAD, possible iatrogenic factors, and in particular chiropractic manipulation of the cervical spine, infection, season, and vascular risk factors.

Activities and Possible Iatrogenic Causes Associated with sCAD

A history of different precipitating events is frequently elicited in patients with sCAD [1]. These events are often characterized by hyperextension, rotation or lateroversion of the neck, and are shown in table 1. Cervical extension and sudden neck movement may both compress the cervical carotid artery against either the transverse processes or the bony mass of the upper three cervical vertebrae or the styloid process of the mastoid bone. The vertebral artery is involved more frequently at the C1–C2 level. Various diagnostic and therapeutic measures may rarely lead to sCAD and are summarized in table 2, whereas complications of chiropractic manipulation of the cervical spine are discussed separately.

Chiropractic Manipulation of the Cervical Spine

Manual cervical spine manipulation is a therapeutic procedure that might result in cerebrovascular insults, primarily due to dissection of the vertebral artery (VAD) [36–38]. This could be due to the anatomy of the vertebral artery which may suffer torsion injury as it curves around the atlas. The artery changes its direction from a vertical path to a horizontal path and is susceptible to injury from rotation and extension [3, 12, 36]. The cervical internal carotid artery is less frequently injured than the vertebral artery during chiropractic maneuvers, probably because it lies freely in the soft tissue of the

Table 1. Activities associated with cervical artery dissection

Sneezing, coughing, vomiting [1, 4, 5]
Intercourse [1, 6]
Extension of the neck over a hairdresser's sink [7, 8]
Rotation of head/neck (abrupt and of short duration or prolonged) [1, 9–14]
Prolonged telephone usage with sustained head rotation and lateroversion [11, 15, 16]
Sport and recreational activities (volleyball, football, wrestling, judo, biking, bowling, trampoline exercises, snow and water skiing, tennis, inline skating, use of roller coaster, golf, yoga, dancing associated with excessive neck movements, painting a ceiling) [9, 13, 17–22]
Carring a heavy burden [23]
Pregnancy and delivery [24, 25]

Table 2. Possible iatrogenic causes of cervical artery dissection

Chiropractic maneuvers [1, 26]
Resuscitation, endotracheal intubation, positioning of neck during anesthesia [27, 28]
Tonsil surgery, tooth extraction on a dental chair [1, 22]
Bronchoscopy, rigid esophagoscopy [28, 29]
Carotid angiography, angioplasty and endarterectomy, intravascular catheter placement [28, 30–33]
Cardiac surgery [28]
Cervical discectomy [34]
Frequent injections of human chorionic gonadotropin and menopausal gonadotropin [35]

neck and is thus more mobile. It is assumed that internal carotid artery dissection during chiropractic manipulation results from compression of the artery against either the transverse processes or the bony mass of the upper cervical vertebrae.

Every year, approximately 250 million chiropractic office visits are carried out in the United States and another 25 million in Canada, and 70% of the visits are for cervical manipulation [39]. Thus, physicians need to be aware of the possible complications related to this therapy.

Several reports and case-control studies have associated chiropractic manipulation of the neck and sCAD [3, 10, 18, 26, 33, 36, 37, 40–46]. The first case of VAD due to chiropractic manipulation was described in 1947 [40]. Previous studies have suggested stroke rates ranging from one in 100,000 to one in 2,000,000 cervical manipulations [26, 39, 44]. Recently, a large population-based, nested case-control study in Ontario, Canada, found a positive association between VAD or occlusion and chiropractic manipulation in young adults younger than 45 years of age, but not for older patients [44]. Since younger people are more likely to have dissection as a cause of stroke [47] and are more likely to visit a chiropractor [48], age should be considered as a possible confounding factor in the above-mentioned study. Smith et al. [26] identified patients with dissection and vertebrobasilar stroke from a prospective stroke registry and assigned stroke etiology in a blind and systematic fashion. The authors compared controls matched for age and sex from the same registry, and interviewed all subjects to determine the timings of both neck pain and cervical manipulation. In multivariate analysis, VAD was independently associated with spinal manipulative therapy within 30 days (OR 6.62; 95% CI 1.4–30). However, patients treated with cervical manipulation showed a trend to be younger than the controls [26].

Efforts to identify patients at risk of sCAD during spinal manipulative therapy, and the type of manipulation most likely to lead to this complication, have not been successful [36–38]. One reason is that most current data are based on retrospective studies. Furthermore, the existing studies have dealt with a low number of events, which impacts the relative risk estimates, because the CI around the risk estimate is very large [46]. In an attempt to resolve the aforementioned problems, Haldeman et al. [18] performed a retrospective review of 64 medicolegal cases of stroke temporally associated with cervical manipulation. At presentation, 92% of cases reported a history of headache and/or neck pain, and 25% complained about the sudden onset of new and unusual head and neck pain often associated with other neurological symptoms such as visual disturbance, dizziness, vertigo, tinnitus, nausea, or vomiting [18]. The remaining patients underwent chiropractic treatment for chronic head or neck pain and some of them had already been treated with chiropractic manipulation. There was no relationship seen between the type of chiropractic manipulation and risk of stroke, as stroke symptoms were reported to begin immediately after the first manipulation or several treatments. The authors found no relation between the number of chiropractic manipulations and the incidence of CAD. The strokes occurred after any form of standard cervical manipulation technique including rotation, extension, lateral flexion, and nonforce and neutral position manipulations. The conclusion of Haldeman et al. [18] was that sCAD and especially VAD should be regarded as a random and unpredictable complication of any neck movement, including cervical manipulation. Thus, a significant increase in pain, especially when associated with focal neurological signs, following spinal manipulative therapy warrants immediate medical evaluation.

Infection

Among other environmental factors, recent infection has been suggested as a possible trigger of endothelial damage and sCAD [2, 49]. Indeed, Grau et al. [56] found a relationship between a recent history of infection and sCAD, comparing 43 patients with sCAD and 58 consecutive ischemic stroke patients younger than 50 years of age. Recent infection was more common in patients with sCAD (58.1%) than in control patients (32.8%, $p = 0.01$). Infection was independently associated with sCAD in the multivariate analysis. Respiratory tract infection was preponderant in both groups [2]. In a subgroup of sCAD patients skin biopsy was performed in order to detect ultrastructural alteration with electron microscopic studies [50]. Patients with pathological findings tended to have more infections than patients without.

In another hospital-based case-control study, Guillon et al. [49] found a higher frequency of infection in patients with sCAD (31.9%) compared to patients with ischemic stroke due to other causes (13.5%). This association was higher in patients with multiple dissections (OR 6.4; 95% CI 0.7–6.3) than in single dissection (OR 2.1; 95% CI 1.7–24). The limitation of this study was that the presence of infection was assessed by a questionnaire and no serological analysis was performed.

It is still unclear how recent infection leads to sCAD. Direct vessel wall injury by a microbial agent and cellular infiltration seems unlikely [51, 52]. The role of indirect inflammatory and immunological host response, with activation of cytokines and proteases could induce excessive extracellular matrix degradation and thus weaken the vessel wall [53, 54]. It is also possible that an underlying asymptomatic structural defect of the arterial wall could predispose to dissection in case an infection is added. These structural defects are often underestimated. Indeed, Goldstein et al. [55] described a young adult whose carotid artery was found to have areas of previous, recurrent dissections as well as an acute lesion, necessitating excision of a pseudoaneurysm. Although there was no angiographic evidence of an arterial anomaly, microscopic evaluation revealed underlying fibromuscular dysplasia. On the other hand mechanical factors associated with infection, such as violent coughing, sneezing, or vomiting, could be responsible for the endothelial tear. This means that in case of infection a minor trauma could also be responsible for sCAD.

Seasonality

A seasonal pattern in the incidence of sCAD was described, suggesting that an environmental factor could lead to sCAD [56]. Schievink et al. [57]

observed this seasonal pattern with a peak in October ($p < 0.02$) in 200 consecutive sCAD patients referred to the Mayo Clinic from 1970 to 1990. The seasonal variation was substantial, with approximately 58% more patients suffering a sCAD in autumn than during other seasons. These results were confirmed also by a subanalysis of patients living within 500 km of the same community (Rochester) in order to avoid the bias of the large climatic fluctuation occurring in Minnesota (USA) ($p < 0.05$). Numerous theories have been proposed to explain the seasonal variations in sCAD, including weather-related changes in blood pressure, coagulation parameters, rheological factors, physical activities, diet, and air pollution [58–60]. Indeed, the seasonal variation of blood pressure is well known, with blood pressure being higher in cold seasons [61] because of a possible cold-induced peripheral blood vessel constriction [43]. However, it is not possible to exclude that cold seasons could favor upper respiratory infections and the above-mentioned minor trauma like sneezing and coughing.

Conventional Vascular Risk Factors

A potential link between conventional vascular risk factors, such as smoking, hypertension, and oral contraceptive use, has not been studied systematically [1]. Pezzini et al. [62] found a higher prevalence of hypertension in patients with sCAD compared to matched controls. In another study the presence of hypertension was associated with a lack of recanalization [63].

Baumgartner et al. [64] observed a higher prevalence of hypercholesterolemia in patients with carotid artery dissection and ischemia, compared to those without ischemia. Because patients with sCAD have by definition no, or at best mild, atherosclerosis, the question arises whether the dissected carotid arteries had also endothelial dysfunction, which might have enhanced thrombus formation and thromboembolism [64].

Hyperhomocysteinemia has also been associated with sCAD as another vascular risk factor [65–67]. However, atherosclerotic vessel lesions are uncommon in sCAD patients [68], thus the role of conventional vascular risk factors seems to be more marginal. Additionally, recurrence of sCAD is rare (0.3% risk per year) [69] compared to atherosclerotic diseases.

Migraine has been shown to be an independent risk factor for sCAD in a case-control study [70]. The authors suggested that the possible underlying arterial wall disease leading to dissection could be a predisposing factor for migraine [71].

Conclusions

The role of environmental factors in the pathogenesis of sCAD is still unclear. The above-mentioned precipitating events often occur in daily life, while sCAD tends to be a unique episode during life. Moreover, sCAD happens especially in patients less than 50 years of age. Maybe, young people are more agile and tend to have more physical activities compared to older patients, but on the other hand vessel walls tend to be more fragile with age. Probably, we are still missing a link between structural defects of the arterial wall and environmental factors leading to sCAD.

References

1 Schievink WI: Spontaneous dissection of the carotid and vertebral arteries. N Engl J Med 2001; 344:899–906.
2 Norris JW, Beletsky V: Carotid dissection and viral illness. Arch Neurol 2000;57:1658–1659.
3 Norris JW, Beletsky V, Nadareishvili ZG: The Canadian Stroke Consortium. Sudden neck movement and cervical artery dissection. CMAJ 2000;163:38–40.
4 Gutowski NJ, Murphy RP, Beale DJ: Unilateral upper cervical posterior spinal artery syndrome following sneezing. J Neurol Neurosurg Psychiatry 1992;55:841–843.
5 Herr RD, Call G, Banks D: Vertebral artery dissection from neck flexion during paroxysmal coughing. Ann Emerg Med 1992;21:88–91.
6 Chang GY, Ahn PC: Postcoital vertebral artery dissection. Am Fam Physician 1996;54: 2195–2196.
7 Weintraub MI: Beauty parlor stroke syndrome: Report of five cases. JAMA 1993;269:2085–2086.
8 Nwokolo N, Bateman DE: Stroke after a visit to the hairdresser. Lancet 1997;350:866.
9 DeBehnke DJ, Brady W: Vertebral artery dissection due to minor neck trauma. J Emerg Med 1994;12:27–31.
10 Frisoni GB, Anzola GP: Vertebrobasilar ischemia after neck motion. Stroke 1991;22:1452–1460.
11 Pryse-Phillips W: Infarction of the medulla and cervical cord after fitness exercises. Stroke 1989;20:292–294.
12 Sherman DG, Hart RG, Easton JD: Abrupt change in head position and cerebral infarction. Stroke 1981;12:2–6.
13 Taniguchi A, Wako K, Naito Y, Kuzuhara S: Wallenberg syndrome and vertebral artery dissection probably due to trivial trauma during golf exercise. Rinsho Shinkeigaku 1993;33:338–340.
14 Traflet RF, Babaria AR, Bell RD, Sollenberger SE, Doan HT, Gonzalez CF, Mishkin MM: Vertebral artery dissection after rapid head turning. AJNR Am J Neuroradiol 1989;10:650–651.
15 Mourad JJ, Girerd X, Safar M: Carotid-artery dissection after a prolonged telephone call. N Engl J Med 1997;336:516.
16 Zuber M, Meder JF, Mas JL: Carotid artery dissection due to elongated styloid process. Neurology 1999;53:1886–1887.
17 Biousse V, Chabriat H, Amarenco P, Bousser MG: Roller-coaster-induced vertebral artery dissection. Lancet 1995;346:767.
18 Haldeman S, Kohlbeck FJ, McGregor M: Stroke, cervical artery dissection, and cervical spine manipulation therapy. J Neurol 2002;249:1098–1104.
19 Hart RG, Easton JD: Dissection of cervical and cerebral arteries. Neurol Clin 1983;1:155–182.
20 Karnik R, Rothmund T, Bonner G, Valentin A, Reuther G: Inline skating as a possible cause of consecutive bilateral vertebral artery dissection. Acta Neurol Scand 2000;101:70–77.

21 Lannuzel A, Moulin T, Amsallem D, Galmiche J, Rumbach L: Vertebral-artery dissection following a judo session: A case report. Neuropediatrics 1994;25:106–108.
22 Prabhakar S, Bhatia R, Khandelwal N, Lal V, Das CP: Vertebral artery dissection due to indirect neck trauma: An underrecognised entity. Neurol India 2001;49:384–390.
23 Bassi P, Lattuada P, Gomitoni A: Cervical cerebral artery dissection: A multicenter prospective study (preliminary report). Neurol Sci 2003;24(suppl 1):S4–S7.
24 Mass SB, Cardonick E, Haas S, Gopalani S, Leuzzi RA: Bilateral vertebral artery dissection causing a cerebrovascular accident in pregnancy. A case report. J Reprod Med 1999;44:887–890.
25 Oehler J, Lichy C, Gandjour J, Fiebach J, Grau AJ: Dissection of four cerebral arteries after protracted birth. Nervenarzt 2003;74:366–369.
26 Smith WS, Johnston SC, Skalabrin EJ, Weaver M, Azari P, Albers GW, Gress DR: Spinal manipulative therapy is an independent risk factor for vertebral artery dissection. Neurology 2003; 60:1424–1428.
27 Rakotoharinandrasana H, Petit E, Dumas P, Vandermarcq P, Gil R, Neau JP: Internal carotid artery dissection after Heimlich maneuver. Ann Fr Anesth Reanim 2003;22:43–45.
28 Adams HP Jr, Love BB, Jacoby MR: Arterial dissections; in Ginsberg MD, Bogousslavsky J (eds): Cerbrovascular Disease: Pathophysiology, Diagnosis and Management. Malden, Blackwell Science, 1998, pp 1430–1445.
29 Ricchetti A, Becker M, Dulguerov P: Internal carotid artery dissection following rigid esophagoscopy. Arch Otolaryngol Head Neck Surg 1999;125:805–807.
30 Braunstein H: Dissecting aneurysm of the carotid artery after carotid angiography. Am Heart J 1964;67:545–549.
31 Davis JM, Zimmerman RA: Injury of the carotid and vertebral arteries. Neuroradiology 1983; 25:55–69.
32 Loftus CM, Dyste GN, Reinarz SJ, Hingtgen WL: Distal cervical carotid dissection after carotid endarterectomy: A complication of indwelling shunt? Neurosurgery 1986;19:441–445.
33 Yu NR, Eberhardt RT, Menzoian JO, Urick CL, Raffetto JD: Vertebral artery dissection following intravascular catheter placement: A case report and review of the literature. Vasc Med 2004;9: 199–203.
34 Manaouil C, Graser M, Delcour J, Le Gars D, Gontier MF, Loriau J, Jarde O: Postoperative bilateral vertebral artery dissection: A case report. J Clin Forensic Med 2003;10:81–84.
35 Wakino S, Tawarahara K, Tsuchiya N, Kurosawa Y, Sugihara T, Ando K: Spontaneous multiple arterial dissections presenting with renal infarction and subarachnoid hemorrhage in a patient under treatment for infertility. Circ J 2005;69:368–372.
36 Assendelft WJ, Bouter LM, Knipschild PG: Complication of spinal manipulation: A comprehensive review of the literature. J Fam Pract 1996;42:475–480.
37 Haldeman S, Kohlbeck FJ, McGregor M: Risk factors and precipitating neck movements causing vertebrobasilar dissection after cervical trauma and spinal manipulation. Spine 1999;24: 785–794.
38 Hart RG, Easton JD: Vertebral artery dissection (editorial). Neurology 1988;38:987–989.
39 Hurwitz EL, Coulter ID, Adams AH, Genovese BJ, Shekelle PG: Use of chiropractic services from 1985 through 1991 in the United States and Canada. Am J Public Health 1998;88:771–776.
40 Bratt-Thomas HR, Berger HR: Cerebellar and spinal injuries after chiropractic manipulation. JAMA 1947;133:600–603.
41 Frumkin LR, Baloh RW: Wallenberg's syndrome following neck manipulation. Neurology 1990;40:611–615.
42 Hufnagel A, Hammers A, Schonle P-W, Bohm K-D, Leonhardt G: Stroke following chiropractic manipulation of the cervical spine. J Neurol 1999;246:683–688.
43 Mas JL, Bousser MG, Hasboun D, Laplane D: Extracranial vertebral artery dissections: A review of 13 cases. Stroke 1987;18:1037–1047.
44 Rothwell DM, Bondy SJ, Williams JI: Chiropractic manipulation and stroke: A population-based case-control study. Stroke 2001;32:1054–1060.
45 Saeed AB, Shuaib A, Al-Sulaiti G, Emery D: Vertebral artery dissection: Warning symptoms, clinical features and prognosis in 26 patients. Can J Neurol Sci 2000;27:292–296.

46 Williams S, Biller J: Vertebrobasilar dissection and cervical spine manipulation. Neurology 2003;60:1408–1409.

47 Bogousslavsky J, Despland PA, Regli F: Spontaneous carotid dissection with acute stroke. Arch Neurol 1987;44:137–140.

48 Coulter ID, Hurwitz EI, Adams AH, Benovese BJ, Hays R, Shekelle PG: Patients using chiropractors in North America: Who are they, and why are they in chiropractic care? Spine 2002; 27:291–296.

49 Guillon B, Berthet K, Benslamia L, Bertrand M, Bousser MG, Tzourio C: Infection and the risk of spontaneous cervical artery dissection. A case-control study. Stroke 2003;34:e79–e81.

50 Brandt T, Hausser I, Orberk E, Grau A, Hartschuh W, Anton-Lamprecht I, Hacke W: Ultrastructural connective tissue abnormalities in patients with spontaneous cervico-cerebral artery dissections. Ann Neurol 1998;44:281–285.

51 Leu HJ: Cerebrovascular accidents resulting from segmental mediolytic arteriopathy of the cerebral arteries in young adults. Cardiovasc Surg 1994;2:350–353.

52 O'Connell BK, Towfighi J, Brennan RW, Tyler W, Mathews M, Weidner WA, Saul RF: Dissecting aneurysms of heart and neck. Neurology 1985;35:993–997.

53 Pober JS: Cytokine-mediated activation of vascular endothelium: Physiology and pathology. Am J Physiol 1988;133:426–433.

54 Smedly LA, Tonnesen MG, Sandhaus RA, Haslett C, Guthrie LA, Johnston RB Jr, Henson PM, Worthen GS: Neutrophil-mediated injury to endothelial cells: Enhancement by endotoxin and essential role of neutrophil elastase. J Clin Invest 1986;77:1233–1243.

55 Goldstein LB, Gray L, Hulette CM: Stroke due to recurrent ipsilateral carotid artery dissection in a young adult. Stroke 1995;26:480–483.

56 Grau AJ, Brandt T, Buggle F, Orberk E, Mytilineos J, Werle E, Conradt C, Krause M, Winter R, Hacke W: Association of cervical artery dissection with recent infection. Arch Neurol 1999;56: 851–856.

57 Schievink WI, Wijdicks EFM, Kuiper JD: Seasonal pattern of spontaneous cervical artery dissection. J Neurosurg 1998;89:101–103.

58 Stout RW, Crawford V: Seasonal variations in fibrinogen concentrations among elderly people. Lancet 1991;338:9–13.

59 Wilmshurst P: Temperature and cardiovascular mortality. Excess deaths from heart disease and stroke in northern Europe are due in part to the cold. Br Med J 1994;309:1029–1030.

60 Woodhouse P, Khaw K-T, Plummer M: Seasonal variation in blood pressure and its relation to ambient temperature in an elderly population. J Hypertens 1983;11:1267.

61 Brennan PJ, Greenberg G, Miall WE, Thompson SG: Seasonal variation in arterial blood pressure. Br Med J 1982;285:919–923.

62 Pezzini A, Caso V, Zanferrari C, Del Zotto E, Paciaroni M, Bartolmo C, Grassi M, Agnelli G, Padovani A: Arterial hypertension as risk factor for cervical artery dissection: A case-control study. JNNP 2005; in press.

63 Caso V, Paciaroni M, Corea F, Hamam M, Milia P, Pelliccioli GP, Parnetti L, Gallai V: Recanalization of cervical artery dissection: Influencing factors and role in neurological outcome. Cerebrovasc Dis 2004;17:93–97.

64 Baumgartner RW, Arnold M, Baumgartner I, Mosso M, Gönner F, Studer A, Schroth G, Schuknecht B, Sturzenegger M: Carotid dissection with and without ischemic events: Local symptoms and cerebral artery findings. Neurology 2001;57:827–832.

65 Caso V, Gallai V: Why should mild hyperhomocysteinemia be responsible for CAD? Stroke 2003;34:209.

66 Gallai V, Caso V, Paciaroni M, Cardioli G, Arning E, Bottiglieri T, Parnetti L: Mild hyperhomocysteinemia: A possible risk factor for cervical artery dissection. Stroke 2001;32:714–718.

67 Pezzini A, Del Zotto E, Archetti S, Negrini R, Bani P, Albertini A, Grassi M, Assanelli D, Gasparotti R, Vignolo LA, Magoni M, Padovani A: Plasma homocysteine concentration, C677T MTHFR genotype, and 844ins68bp CBS genotype in young adults with spontaneous cervical artery dissection and atherothrombotic stroke. Stroke 2002;33:664–669.

68 Mokri B, Sundt TMJ, Houser OW, Piepgras DW: Spontaneous dissection of the cervical internal carotid artery. Ann Neurol 1986;19:126–138.

69 Touzé E, Gauvrit JY, Moulin T, Meder JF, Bracard S, Mas JL, for the Multicenter Survey on Natural History of Cervical Artery Dissection: Risk of stroke and recurrent dissection after a cervical artery dissection. A multicenter study. Neurology 2003;61:1347–1351.
70 D'Anglejan-Chatillon J, Ribeiro V, Mas JL, Youl BD, Bousser MG. Migraine – A risk factor for dissection of cervical arteries. Headache 1989;29:560–561.
71 Tzourio C, Benslamia L, Guillon B, Aidi S, Bertrand M, Berthet K, Bousser MG: Migraine and the risk of cervical artery dissection: A case-control study. Neurology 2002;59:435–437.

Dr. Dr. Valeria Caso
Department of Neuroscience
University of Perugia
Via Enrico dal Pozzo, IT–06126 Perugia (Italy)
Tel. +39 075 578 3970, Fax +39 075 578 3870, E-Mail vcaso@hotmail.com

Baumgartner RW, Bogousslavsky J, Caso V, Paciaroni M (eds): Handbook on Cerebral Artery Dissection. Front Neurol Neurosci. Basel, Karger, 2005, vol 20, pp 54–63

Traumatic Cervical Artery Dissection

Krassen Nedeltchev[a], *Ralf W. Baumgartner*[b]

[a]Institute of Diagnostic and Interventional Neuroradiology, University Hospital of Bern, Bern, and [b]Department of Neurology, University Hospital of Zürich, Zürich, Switzerland

Abstract

Traumatic cervical artery dissection (TCAD) is a complication of severe blunt head or neck trauma, the main cause being motor vehicle accidents. TCAD are increasingly recognized, and incidences of up to 0.86% for internal carotid and 0.53% for traumatic vertebral artery dissections (TVAD) among blunt trauma victims are reported. Diagnostic evaluation for TCAD is mandatory in the presence of (1) hemorrhage of potential arterial origin originating from the nose, ears, mouth, or a wound; (2) expanding cervical hematoma; (3) cervical bruit in a patient >50 years of age; (4) evidence of acute infarct at brain imaging; (5) unexplained central or lateralizing neurological deficit or transient ischemic attack, or (6) Horner syndrome, neck or head pain. In addition, a number of centers screen asymptomatic patients with blunt trauma for TCAD. Catheter angiography is the standard of reference for diagnosis of TCAD. Color duplex ultrasound, computed tomographic, and magnetic resonance angiography are noninvasive screening alternatives, but each method has its diagnostic limitations compared to catheter angiography. Anticoagulants and antiplatelet drugs may prevent ischemic stroke, but bleeding from traumatized tissues may offset the benefits of antithrombotic treatment. Endovascular therapy of dissected vessels, thrombarterectomy, direct suture of intimal tears, and extracranial–intracranial bypass should be considered in exceptional cases. Neurological outcome is probably worse in TCAD compared to spontaneous CAD, although it is unclear whether this is due to dissection-induced ischemic stroke or associated traumatic lesions.

Cervical artery dissection (CAD) is considered to be either traumatic (TCAD) or spontaneous in origin. TCAD mainly complicates severe blunt head or neck traumas, which are most often due to motor vehicle accidents. Conversely, spontaneous CAD occurs without a precipitating event or may be preceded by a so-called minor trauma. A minor trauma is an event, which is generally not followed by CAD (e.g. sneezing, coughing, vomiting, sport, and recreational activities), and is discussed in the chapter by Caso et al. (pp. 44–53). Iatrogenic CAD is a special subgroup of minor trauma, because it is an exceptional complication of diagnostic and therapeutic interventions. Nevertheless, the classification of CAD into traumatic and spontaneous forms may be arbitrary in some cases.

Traumatologists also coined the term 'blunt cerebrovascular injury' (BCVI) for patients who developed lesions of the carotid (BCI) or vertebral (BVI) artery after a blunt trauma [1]. Biffl et al. [2] used a 5-grade scale to classify angiographic lesions to describe BCVI, suggesting that CAD is not always the consequence of BCVI. However, Biffl et al. [3] state that the etiology of BCVI is an intimal tear. Thus, the term TCAD will be used as synonym for BCVI, traumatic internal carotid artery dissection (TICAD) for BCI, and traumatic vertebral artery dissection (TVAD) for BVI.

Epidemiology

BCI was first described in 1872, and there were only 96 cases reported up to 1980 [4]. Studies performed in the late 1980s reported an incidence of 0.08% [1]. In the 1990s, the awareness of the potentially severe complications of TCAD and the recognition of BCVI distinct from head injury augmented, and a raising number of centers introduced screening protocols for asymptomatic patients with blunt trauma [5]. Subsequent investigations have detected more patients with TICAD leading to incidences of up to 0.5% for all blunt trauma patients, and up to 0.67% for motor vehicle accident victims [1, 6, 7]. The largest published series to date comprised 18,233 patients with blunt trauma and described what the authors called the unrecognized epidemic of BCI [8]. The first retrospective part of the study covered a period of 6 years and reported a 0.1% incidence of BCI. The subsequent prospective second part lasted for 2.5 years and yielded a 0.86% BCI rate. Carotid dissection, alone or in combination with pseudoaneurysm, carotid artery occlusion or carotid-cavernous sinus fistula, was present in 84% of the patients. A more recent study evaluated retrospectively the medical records of 3,342 patients admitted to a trauma center during a period of 3 years [9]. The incidence of TICAD was 0.21% for all trauma patients. When examining those patients who were more severely injured and at risk for occult carotid artery injury, the incidence of TICAD increased to 3.2%. Screening patients based on injury mechanisms and patterns for TVAD detected an incidence of 0.53% [10]. Recent evidence indicates that vertebral artery (VA) injury may be very common in conjunction with certain injury patterns [10, 11].

Etiology

The main cause of TCAD is motor vehicle collision [6, 8, 12]. Furthermore, patients with combinations of head, facial, and cervical spine injuries are at increased risk for TCAD. Basilar skull fracture, and especially fracture through the petrous segment of the carotid canal, bears a significant risk of carotid injury [13]. Injuries of the VA occur usually without fractures or dislocations. However, Willis et al. [14] described several patients with unstable cervical fractures affecting also the transversal foramina, who presented in 46% asymptomatic TVAD.

Pathogenesis of TCAD

In 1974, Crissey and Bernstein [15] described four mechanisms leading to injury of the cervical ICA: (1) direct blow to the neck, (2) neck hyperextension associated with rotation, (3) blunt intraoral trauma, and (4) basilar skull fracture involving the carotid canal. Direct blow to the neck was responsible for up to 50% of cases in this report. Subsequent studies emphasized the role of the second mechanism, neck hyperextension with rotation, which are particularly common in motor vehicle accidents [16]. The aforementioned neck movements may also press the cervical carotid artery against the lateral mass of either C1 or C2. The third mechanism is characteristic for children, who fall with an object such as a pencil or toothbrush in the mouth. The forth mechanism, basilar skull fracture, seems to provide a relevant source of unrecognized carotid artery injuries [17]. Kerwin et al. [18] performed 4-vessel angiography in 48 patients with blunt trauma, who were thought to be at high risk for BCI. Sixty percent of all patients with basilar skull fractures who were otherwise asymptomatic had abnormal angiograms.

The VA is most susceptible to injury at the point of entrance into the foramen transversarium C6. The artery is relatively fixed at the bony orifice of the foramen, and the increased mobility at C5/6 makes it vulnerable. The rotation in the atlantoaxial joint and the flexion/extension in the atlanto-occipital joint designate the second most common site of TVAD at C1–C2 [19, 20].

Neurological Manifestations

The neurological manifestations of TCAD and spontaneous CAD do not differ and are discussed in the chapters by Baumgartner and Bogousslavsky (pp. 70–76), and Arnold and Bousser (pp. 77–86). It is unclear whether clinical signs and symptoms occur with different frequency in TCAD compared to spontaneous CAD.

Diagnosis

A diagnostic evaluation for TCAD is mandatory, if emergent diagnostic testing shows signs or symptoms of BCVI mentioned below [5]. In addition, the results of several studies have led to the development of protocols for the screening of asymptomatic patients without signs and symptoms of cerebrovascular injury for the presence of TCAD.

Signs and symptoms of BCVI are an indication for a diagnostic work-up of the cerebral arteries in order to detect TCAD, and include: (1) hemorrhage of potential arterial origin originating from the nose, ears, mouth, or a wound; (2) expanding cervical hematoma; (3) cervical bruit in a patient older than 50 years of age; (4) evidence of acute infarct at brain imaging; (5) unexplained or CT incongruous central or lateralizing neurological deficit or transient ischemic attack, and (6) Horner syndrome, neck or head pain, although pain may result from other injuries.

The rationale for screening of asymptomatic trauma patients for the presence of TCAD is that (1) BCVI occurs in many asymptomatic patients [21], (2) anticoagulation improves neurological outcome and potentially prevents strokes [6], and (3) in 44% of cases there was an interval of at least 18 h between the time of injury and the onset of ischemic symptoms, during which antithrombotic therapy could be instituted [3]. The screening protocols differ from center to center, and the incidence of TCAD correlates with the criteria applied for screening and the sensitivity of the diagnostic tests, which are shown in table 1. Biffl et al. [22] have recently published a report that attempted to define high-risk groups who should undergo screening angiography to exclude TCAD [22]. Four factors predictive of TCAD were identified: (1) GCS score ≤6, signs of (2) petrous bone fracture, (3) diffuse axonal injury of the brain, or (4) Le Fort II or III fractures at cranial imaging. Furthermore, cervical spine fractures were highly associated with TCAD. Correspondingly, Willis et al. [14] used cervical spine subluxation from a 'locked' or 'perched' facet, facet destruction with evidence of instability, or a fracture involving the foramen transversarium as screening criteria for patients who should undergo catheter angiography to exclude VA injury. In a more recent report, Veras et al. [23] reported 6 cases of VA injury in patients with cervical spine facet joint dislocation or foramen transversarium fractures.

The tests used for diagnosis of TCAD and spontaneous CAD are identical and summarized in the chapters by Benninger et al. (pp. 87–101), Paciaroni et al. (pp. 102–118), and Taschner et al. (pp. 119–128).

Four-vessel biplanar cerebral catheter angiography is the gold standard for diagnosis of TCAD. All four vessels should be imaged from their origins to their terminal branches in order to identify occluded terminal vessels. Unfortunately,

Table 1. Indications for screening arteriography or magnetic resonance angiography and frequency of abnormal findings

Source	Diagnostic test	Reason screened	Incidence
Louw et al. [50]	Arteriography	Cervical spine facet dislocation	9/12 BVI
Willis et al. [14]	Arteriography	Cervical spine subluxation, foramen transversarium fracture	12/26 BVI
Friedman et al. [51]	MRA	C-spine injury	9/37 BVI
Fabian et al. [6]	Arteriography	Neck injury, Horner's syndrome	23% BCI
		Incompatible neurological and CT findings	34% BCI
		New onset of neurological deficits	43% BCI
Giacobetti et al. [52]	MRA	Cervical spine injury	12/61 BVI
Weller et al. [53]	MRA	Foramen transversarium fracture	4/12 BVI
Carrillo et al. [54]	Arteriography/MRA	New onset of neurological deficits	15/30 BCI
		CT findings suggesting BCI	15/30 BCI
Kerwin et al. [18]	Arteriography	Carotid canal, foramen transversarium, flexion/ extension cervical spine, massive facial fracture	1.1%
Parbhoo et al. [55]	MRA	Cervical spine fracture, dislocation	12/47 BVI
Biffl et al. [3]	Arteriography	Hemorrhage of potential arterial origin, expanding cervical hematoma, cervical bruit in a patient older than 50 years of age, acute infarct at brain imaging, incompatible neurological and CT findings, Horner's syndrome	1.55%
Miller et al. [56]	Arteriography	Cervical spine, Le Fort II/III, foramen lacerum fracture, cervical soft tissue injuries	1.03%
Rozycki et al. [57]	Arteriography	Cervicothoracic seat-belt sign	4/131 BCI

BCI = Blunt carotid artery injury, BVI = blunt vertebral artery injury, MRA = magnetic resonance angiography.

catheter angiography is invasive and resource-intensive. Its risks include complications related to catheter insertion and contrast administration (1–2% each) and stroke (less than 1%) [5]. Color duplex ultrasound, computed tomographic and magnetic resonance angiography (MRA) are currently considered reliable noninvasive modalities for screening. The advantages and limitations of these techniques are discussed in the chapters by Benninger et al. (pp. 87–101), Paciaroni et al. (pp. 102–108), and Taschner et al. (pp. 119–128).

Treatment

Anticoagulants and antiplatelet drugs may preclude arterial thrombosis in TCAD, and thus prevent ischemic stroke. With the exception that sequelae of the trauma such as bleeding or consecutive operations may limit the use of the aforementioned antithrombotic agents, the indication and duration of this therapy does not differ from patients with spontaneous CAD and is discussed in the chapter by Engelter and Lyrer (pp. 147–159).

Thromboendarterectomy, direct suture of intimal tears, extracranial–intracranial bypass, and excision of the injured segment with interposition of arterial or venous graft have been performed with varying success [24, 25]. Complications of surgery included stroke, early and delayed graft reocclusion, inability to access the injured segment, and lesions of cranial nerves. The benign clinical course of patients with spontaneous CAD treated with antithrombotic therapy suggests that surgery should be considered in exceptional cases of TCAD [26, 27].

Endovascular treatment is currently an area under vigorous investigation. Coldwell et al. [28] stented 16 pseudoaneurysms in 14 patients and demonstrated resolution of all lesions within 4 months of warfarin therapy. Stents have successfully been deployed in patients with both extra- and intracranial carotid dissections [29, 30]. Taking the benign course of pseudoaneurysm [31, 32], persistent stenosis, and occlusion [33] in patients with spontaneous internal carotid artery dissection into consideration, it seems that a conservative approach of the above-mentioned carotid lesions should be the norm and endovascular therapy the exception, such as cases with vessel rupture and bleeding into the neck.

Intravenous thrombolysis is contraindicated in patients with TCAD. Conversely, local intra-arterial thrombolysis has been successfully used in patients with spontaneous (see chapter by Georgiadis and Baumgartner, (pp. 70–76) and ICAD [34, 35]. However, local intra-arterial thrombolysis is likely to be associated with a certain bleeding risk in injured body parts of patients with TCAD, because the thrombolytic drug may enter cerebral veins. This assumption is underscored by the increased bleeding rate in operated organs and wounds of patients who were treated with local intra-arterial thrombolysis for acute ischemic stroke and underwent major surgery within the preceding few days [36].

Prognosis

Different studies have reported a highly variable course of TCAD. Generally, TCAD seem to have a less favorable outcome than spontaneous ones [37]. The prevalence of permanent neurological deficits range from 40 to 80% [4, 37–39], larger series report mortality rates from 20 to 40% [4, 40, 41]. However, the aforementioned comparison is hampered by the fact that the high morbidity and mortality rates partially result from the accompanying traumatic lesions of the brain and spinal cord. Biffl et al. [2] hypothesized that different grades of cervical artery injury might have distinct implications in terms of response to therapy and neurological outcome. They proposed a grading scale that was based on the angiographic appearance of the injury and divided the carotid artery injuries into five grades: (I) irregularity of the vessel wall or a dissection with <25% luminal stenosis; (II) intraluminal thrombus or raised intimal flap, or dissection or intramural hematoma causing a luminal narrowing >25%; (III) pseudoaneurysm; (IV) vessel occlusion, and (V) vessel transection with free contrast extravasation. At follow-up, a complete angiographic restitution was noted in 68% of the patients with grade I cervical artery injury. Angiographic progression toward a higher grade was observed in 7% of cases. The grade II lesions healed, improved, and persisted in 10% each; 70% of the injuries worsened. Despite angiographic progression, just one patient suffered a stroke, suggesting a benefit in anticoagulation. Eighty-five percent of the pseudoaneurysms (grade III) persisted on follow-up angiography, only one of 16 pseudoaneurysms healed while on heparin. Two internal carotid artery dissections (grade IV) were reimaged after 7–10 days; neither had changed. For comparison, series including spontaneous CAD report recanalization in 68–100% of stenosis and in 25–43% of occlusions [42–47].

A recent study analyzed the neurological outcome of 21 patients with TCAD with regard to the treatment (heparin, n = 12; aspirin 325 mg/day, n = 6; no therapy, n = 3) [18]. The study demonstrated no difference in outcome on the basis of antithrombotic therapy. There were no deaths as a direct result of the vascular injury. There were bleeding complications at the surgical site (n = 3), injury site (n = 2), and in the gastrointestinal tract (n = 1) after initiation of systemic heparin therapy.

Repeated dissection can occur in 0–8% of patients with spontaneous CAD [42–44, 48]. The rate of redissection in TCAD is unknown. Dziewas et al. [49] assessed retrospectively the clinical outcome of 29 patients with TCAD and 97 patients with spontaneous CAD [49]. A recurrent dissection occurred in 4 patients (3.2%) within the first month and in 2 patients (1.6%) within the period of one month to one year, though the authors did not specify the etiology of the inclusion dissection.

Conclusion

TCAD is uncommon, but its incidence is increasing over the last years. Recent progress in neuroimaging and implementation of appropriate screening criteria detected an unprecedented number of cervical artery injuries among patients with blunt head or neck trauma. Cerebral infarction due to distal thrombus embolization is the most relevant clinical manifestation of TCAD. Early recognition of neurovascular trauma and institution of antithrombotic treatment may preclude arterial thrombosis and thus prevent ischemic stroke. However, randomized trials assessing the efficacy of antithrombotic therapy are missing so far. Increased bleeding may offset the benefits of the antithrombotic treatment. Despite treatment, permanent neurological deficits and death are unavoidable in significant proportion of cases.

References

1 Davis JW, Holbrook TL, Hoyt DB, Mackersie RC, Field TOJ, Shackford SR: Blunt carotid artery dissection: Incidence, associated injuries, screening, and treatment. J Trauma 1990;30:1514– 1517.

2 Biffl WL, Moore EE, Offner PJ, Brega KE, Franciose RJ, Burch JM: Blunt carotid arterial injuries: Implications of a new grading scale. J Trauma 1999;47:845–853.

3 Biffl WL, Ray CE Jr, Moore EE, Franciose RJ, Aly S, Heyrose MG, Johnson JL, Burch JM: Treatment-related outcomes from blunt cerebrovascular injuries. Importance of routine follow-up arteriography. Ann Surg 2002;235:699–707.

4 Krajewski LP, Hertzer NR: Blunt carotid artery trauma: Report of two cases and review of the literature. Ann Surg 1980;191:341–346.

5 Biffl WL: Diagnosis of blunt cerebrovascular injuries. Curr Opin Crit Care 2003;9:530–534.

6 Fabian TC, Patton JH Jr, Croce MA, Minard G, Kudsk KA, Pritchard FE: Blunt carotid injury: Importance of early diagnosis and anticoagulant therapy. Ann Surg 1996;223:513–525.

7 Laitt RD, Lewis TT, Bradshaw JR: Blunt carotid arterial trauma. Clin Radiol 1996;51:117–122.

8 Biffl WL, Moore EE, Ryu RK, Offner PJ, Novak Z, Coldwell DM, Franciose RJ, Burch JM: The unrecognized epidemic of blunt carotid arterial injuries: Early diagnosis improves neurologic outcome. Ann Surg 1998;228:462–470.

9 Hughes KM, Collier B, Greene KA, Kurek S: Traumatic carotid artery dissection: A significant incidental finding. Am Surg 2000;66:1023–1027.

10 Miller FB, Fabian TC, Bee TK, Timmons S, Chamsuddin A, Finkle R, Croce MA: Blunt cerebrovascular injuries: Diagnosis and treatment. J Trauma 2001;51:279–285.

11 Biffl WL, Moore EE, Elliott JP, Ray C, Offner PJ, Franciose RJ, Brega KE, Burch JM: The devastating potential of blunt vertebral arterial injuries. Ann Surg 2000;23:672–681.

12 Kraus RR, Bergstein JM, DeBord JR: Diagnosis, treatment, and outcome of blunt carotid arterial injuries. Am J Surg 1999;178:190–193.

13 Resnick DK, Subach BR, Marion DW: The significance of carotid canal involvement in basilar cranial fracture. Neurosurgery 1997;40:1177–1181.

14 Willis BK, Greiner F, Orrison WW, Benzel EC: The incidence of vertebral artery injury after midcervical spine fracture or subluxation. Neurosurgery 1994;34:435–441.

15 Crissey MM, Bernstein EF: Delayed presentation of carotid intimal tear following blunt craniocervical trauma. Surgery 1974;75:543–549.

16 Biffl WL, Moore EE, Offner PJ, Burch JM: Blunt carotid and vertebral arterial injuries. World J Surg 2001;25:1036–1043.

17 Carter DA, Mehelas TJ, Savolaine ER, Dougherty LS: Basal skull fracture with traumatic polycranial neuropathy and occluded left carotid artery: Significance of fractures along the course of the carotid artery. J Trauma 1998;44:230–235.
18 Kerwin AJ, Bynoe RP, Murray J, Hudson ER, Close TP, Gifford RR, Carson KW, Smith LP, Bell RM: Liberalized screening for blunt carotid and vertebral artery injuries is justified. J Trauma 2001;51:308–314.
19 Sheth TN, Winslow JL, Mikulis DJ: Rotational changes in the morphology of the vertebral artery at a common site of artery dissection. Can Assoc Radiol J 2001;52:236–241.
20 Pelkonen O, Tikkakoski T, Leinonen S, Pyhtinen J, Lepojarvi M, Sotaniemi K: Extracranial internal carotid and vertebral artery dissections: Angiographic spectrum, course and prognosis. Neuroradiology 2003;45:71–77.
21 Prall JA, Brega KE, Coldwell DM, Breeze RE: Incidence of unsuspected blunt carotid artery injury. Neurosurgery 1998;42:495–498.
22 Biffl WL, Moore EE, Offner PJ, Brega KE, Franciose RJ, Elliott JP, Burch JM: Optimizing screening for blunt cerebrovascular injuries. Am J Surg 1999;178:517–522.
23 Veras LM, Pedraza-Gutierrez S, Castellanos J, Capellades J, Casamitjana J, Rovira-Canellas A: Vertebral artery occlusion after acute cervical spine trauma. Spine 2000;25:1171–1177.
24 Alimi YS, Di Mauro P, Fiacre E, Magnan J, Juhan C: Blunt injury to the internal carotid artery at the base of the skull: Six cases of venous graft restoration. J Vasc Surg 1996;24:249–257.
25 Muller BT, Luther B, Hort W, Neumann-Haefelin T, Aulich A, Sandmann W: Surgical treatment of 50 carotid dissections: Indications and results. J Vasc Surg 2000;31:980–988.
26 Schievink WI, Mokri B, O'Fallon WM: Recurrent spontaneous cervical artery dissection. N Engl J Med 1994;330:393–397.
27 Touzé E, Gauvrit JY, Moulin T, Meder JF, Bracard S, Mas JL, for the Multicenter Survey on Natural History of Cervical Artery Dissection: Risk of stroke and recurrent dissection after a cervical artery dissection. A multicenter study. Neurology 2003;61:1347–1351.
28 Coldwell DM, Novak Z, Ryu RK, Brega KE, Biffl WL, Offner PJ, Franciose RJ, Burch JM, Moore EE: Treatment of posttraumatic internal carotid arterial pseudoaneurysms with endovascular stents. J Trauma 2000;48:470–472.
29 Hemphill JC 3rd, Gress DR, Halbach VV: Endovascular therapy of traumatic injuries of the intracranial cerebral arteries. Crit Care Clin 1999;15:811–829.
30 Gomez CR, May AK, Terry JB, Tulyapronchote R: Endovascular therapy of traumatic injuries of the extracranial cerebral arteries. Crit Care Clin 1999;15:789–809.
31 Guillon B, Brunerau L, Biousse V, Djouhri H, Lévy C, Bousser MG: Long-term follow-up of aneurysms developed during extracranial internal carotid artery dissection. Neurology 1999;53:117–122.
32 Touzé E, Randoux B, Méary E, Arquizan C, Meder JF, Mas JL: Aneurysmal forms of cervical artery dissection. Associated factors and outcome. Stroke 2001;32:418–423.
33 Kremer C, Mosso M, Georgiadis D, Stöckli E, Benninger D, Arnold M, Baumgartner RW: Carotid dissection with permanent and transient occlusion or severe stenosis: Long-term outcome. Neurology 2003;60:271–275.
34 Price RF, Sellar R, Leung C, O'Sullivan MJ: Traumatic vertebral arterial dissection and vertebrobasilar arterial thrombosis successfully treated with endovascular thrombolysis and stenting. AJNR Am J Neuroradiol 1998;19:1677–1680.
35 Arnold M, Nedeltchev K, Sturzenegger M, Schroth G, Loher TJ, Stepper F, Remonda L, Bassetti C, Mattle HP: Thrombolysis in patients with acute stroke caused by cervical artery dissection: Analysis of 9 patients and review of the literature. Arch Neurol 2002;59:549–553.
36 Chalela JA, Katzan I, Liebeskind DS, Rasmussen P, Zaidat O, Suarez JI, Chiu D, Klucznick RP, Jauch E, Cucchiara BL, Saver J, Kasner SE, Demchuk AM: Safety of intra-arterial thrombolysis in the postoperative period. Stroke 2001;32:1365–1369.
37 Mokri B: Traumatic and spontaneous extracranial internal carotid artery dissections. J Neurol 1990;237:356–361.
38 Yamada S, Kindt GW, Youmans JR: Carotid artery occlusion due to nonpenetrating injury. J Trauma 1967;7:333–342.

39 Mears GD, Leonard RB: Blunt carotid artery trauma: A case report. J Emerg Med 1988;6: 281–284.
40 Perry MO, Snyder WH, Thal ER: Carotid artery injuries caused by blunt trauma. Ann Surg 1980; 192:74–77.
41 Maurer PK, Plassche W, Green RM: Blunt trauma to the carotid artery with transient deficit and early repair. Surg Neurol 1984;21:110–112.
42 Bogousslavsky J, Despland PA, Regli F: Spontaneous carotid dissection with acute stroke. Arch Neurol 1987;44:137–140.
43 Ast G, Woimant F, Georges B, Laurian C, Haguenau M: Spontaneous dissection of the internal carotid artery in 68 patients. Eur J Med 1993;2:466–472.
44 Mokri B, Sundt TMJ, Houser OW, Piepgras DG: Spontaneous dissection of the cervical internal carotid artery. Ann Neurol 1986;19:126–138.
45 Sturzenegger M: Spontaneous internal carotid artery dissection: Early diagnosis and management in 44 patients. J Neurol 1995;242:231–238.
46 Steinke W, Rautenberg W, Schwartz A, Hennerici M: Noninvasive monitoring of internal carotid artery dissection. Stroke 1994;25:998–1005.
47 Petro GR, Witwer GA, Cacayorin ED, Hodge CJ, Bredenberg CE, Jastremski MS, Kieffer SA: Spontaneous dissection of the cervical internal carotid artery: Correlation of arteriography, CT, and pathology. AJR Am J Roentgenol 1987;148:393–398.
48 Schievink WI, Mokri B, Piepgras DG, Kuiper JD: Recurrent spontaneous arterial dissections: Risk in familial versus nonfamilial disease. Stroke 1996;27:622–624.
49 Dziewas R, Konrad C, Drager B, Evers S, Besselmann M, Ludemann P, Kuhlenbaumer G, Stogbauer F, Ringelstein EB: Cervical artery dissection – Clinical features, risk factors, therapy and outcome in 126 patients. J Neurol 2003;250:1179–1184.
50 Louw JA, Mafoyane NA, Small B, Neser CP: Occlusion of the vertebral artery in cervical spine dislocations. J Bone Joint Surg Br 1990;72:679–681.
51 Friedman D, Flanders A, Thomas C, Millar W: Vertebral artery injury after acute cervical spine trauma: Rate of occurrence as detected by MR angiography and assessment of clinical consequences. AJR Am J Roentgenol 1995;164:443–447.
52 Giacobetti FB, Vaccaro AR, Bos-Giacobetti MA, Deeley DM, Albert TJ, Farmer JC, Cotler JM: Vertebral artery occlusion associated with cervical spine trauma. A prospective analysis. Spine 1997;22:188–192.
53 Weller SJ, Rossitch EJ, Malek AM: Detection of vertebral artery injury after cervical spine trauma using magnetic resonance angiography. J Trauma 1999;46:660–666.
54 Carrillo EH, Osborne DL, Spain DA, Miller FB, Senler SO, Richardson JD: Blunt carotid artery injuries: Difficulties with the diagnosis prior to neurologic event. J Trauma 1999;46:1120–1125.
55 Parbhoo AH, Govender S, Corr P: Vertebral artery injury in cervical spine trauma. Injury 2001;32:565–568.
56 Miller PR, Fabian TC, Croce MA, Cagiannos C, Williams JS, Vang M, Qaisi WG, Felker RE, Timmons SD: Prospective screening for blunt cerebrovascular injuries: Analysis of diagnostic modalities and outcomes. Ann Surg 2002;236:386–393.
57 Rozycki GS, Tremblay L, Feliciano DV, Tchorz K, Hattaway A, Fountain J, Pettitt BJ: A prospective study for the detection of vascular injury in adult and pediatric patients with cervicothoracic seat belt signs. J Trauma 2002;52:618–623.

Dr. Krassen Nedeltchev
Department of Neurology, University Hospital of Bern
Inselspital
CH–3010 Bern (Switzerland)
Tel. +41 31 632 9522, Fax +41 31 632 4872, E-Mail krassen.nedeltchev@insel.ch

Baumgartner RW, Bogousslavsky J, Caso V, Paciaroni M (eds): Handbook on Cerebral Artery Dissection. Front Neurol Neurosci. Basel, Karger, 2005, vol 20, pp 64–69

Vasodilation in Spontaneous Cervical Artery Dissection

C. Lucas, D. Leys

Department of Neurology, Lille University Hospital, Lille, France

Abstract

Cervical artery dissection (CAD) accounts for 10–20% of ischemic strokes in young adults. Although trauma and pre-existing disorders of the arterial wall are the main predisposing factors, most CAD are considered as 'spontaneous'. We hypothesized that CAD could originate in a systemic vascular disease, bound to the intima–media interface, with no clinical sign. If this hypothesis is true, the endothelium-dependent vasodilation would be impaired in response to physiological stimulus such as blood flow increase. Flow-mediated arterial dilation was studied in 65 consecutive patients with spontaneous CAD: 26 with internal carotid artery dissection (ICAD), and 39 with vertebral artery dissection (VAD) were included. CAD patients with vascular risk factors, trivial or obvious cervical trauma, or connective tissue disease were excluded. Twenty-three patients with ischemic stroke of unknown cause were included as controls. Using high-resolution ultrasonography, brachial artery diameter was measured at rest, during postischemic hyperemia (flow-mediated endothelium-dependent dilation), and after sublingual glyceryl trinitrate spray (endothelium-independent dilation). The means (SD) of flow-mediated vasodilation index were 5.7% (6.2) in ICAD, 5.0% (9.3) in VAD, and 13.2% (6.5) in controls ($p < 0.0005$), without any difference between ICAD and VAD; endothelium-independent dilation means were 21.5% (9.5) in ICAD, 25.1% (12.5) in VAD, and 20.8% (8.4) in controls, without significant difference between groups ($p = 0.49$). These results give evidence for an impaired endothelium-dependent vasodilation in CAD patients that is not the consequence of stroke and suggest that an underlying abnormality of the arterial wall layers may predispose to CAD.

A cervical trauma can be a triggering factor for cervical artery dissection (CAD) [1, 2], but a history of trauma is absent in many patients, leading to the concept of 'spontaneous' CAD [3, 4]. Concomitant dissections of cervical and renal arteries [5], an increased diameter of the aortic arch in patients with spontaneous CAD [6], and modifications of carotid wall properties [7] support the hypothesis that an asymptomatic general vascular disorder of the arterial wall may predispose to CAD. Guillon et al. [7] have compared the hemodynamic and morphological properties of carotid arteries in 26 patients with spontaneous internal carotid artery dissection (ICAD) and 26 controls matched for age, sex, and height. Patients and controls had ultrasound measurement of common carotid artery diameter, and diameter changes during the cardiac cycle, bulbar and suprabulbar internal carotid artery diameters, and common carotid artery intima–media thickness. The unaffected carotid artery in patients was compared with the carotid artery of the same side in controls. Common carotid artery relative diameter changes were significantly higher in patients than controls, whereas other measurements did not significantly differ between both groups. In multivariate analyses, the highest tertile of common carotid artery relative diameter changes was associated with the risk of ICAD (OR, 10.0; 95% CI, 1.8–54.2; $p = 0.002$). Therefore, an underlying arteriopathy, presumably related to an extracellular matrix defect, is likely to be present in patients with spontaneous ICAD.

Endothelium and Vascular Diseases

The endothelium is responsible for a powerful local active vasodilation [8, 9] that can be induced by physiological stimuli such as blood flow. Under physiological conditions most vessels react to an increased blood flow and increased shear stress by an increase in diameter [10]. It has been shown that the so-called flow-mediated vasodilation (FMD) is endothelium dependent, and mainly due to nitric oxide (NO) release by endothelial cells [11]. NO production is initiated by the effect of shear stress on the endothelial cell [12]. This property is impaired in patients with vascular risk factors such as smoking [14, 17], arterial hypertension [15], diabetes mellitus [22], or hypercholesterolemia [16, 19]. Moreover, the impairment of the endothelium function occurs a long time before the appearance of clinical signs, suggesting that early subtle damages of the arterial wall may induce significant changes in endothelial response. Therefore, mild endothelial dysfunction, irrespective of its origin, can be revealed by examining the efficiency of a blood flow alteration to change the diameter of blood vessels. In humans, FMD can be simply achieved by postischemic hyperemia induced in the brachial artery [13, 19–21].

Vasoreactivity, Endothelium Function and CAD

For the aforementioned reasons, we tested the hypothesis that endothelial function is impaired in patients with spontaneous CAD [18]. FMD was studied

Table 1. Study population. Number, sex, age, and period between ischemic stroke and vasoreactivity test (PED) in patients with internal carotid artery dissection (ICAD), vertebral artery dissection (VAD), and controls

	ICAD	VAD	Controls	p*
N (men/women)	26 (17/9)	39 (17/22)	23 (11/12)	0.216
Mean age (SD) (years)	41.8 (8.06)	45.6 (7.73)	43.6 (9.26)	0.186
PED (days)	664 (556)	866 (658)	1087 (538)	0.043

*p values have been obtained with the Kruskal-Wallis test.

in 65 consecutive patients with spontaneous CAD including 26 cases with ICAD and 39 cases with vertebral artery dissection (VAD). We excluded CAD patients with vascular risk factors, trivial or obvious cervical trauma, or connective tissue disease. Twenty-three patients with ischemic stroke of unknown cause were included as controls. The endothelium reactivity test was done at least 80 days after the ischemic stroke to avoid a potential effect of the stroke itself on vascular function (table 1). Using high-resolution ultrasonography, brachial artery diameter was measured at rest, during postischemic hyperemia (flow-mediated endothelium-dependent dilation), and after sublingual administration of glyceryl trinitrate (GTN) spray (endothelium-independent dilation). Distal ischemia was obtained by inflating a pneumatic cuff placed around the forearm, to about 40 mm Hg above the systolic pressure, for 3 min [16]. The artery was scanned for 1 min before inflation to measure the artery diameter at rest (d_0), and 2 min after deflation, to measure the maximal diameter during hyperemia (d_h). The endothelium-dependent vasodilation was assessed by calculating the flow-mediated index (FMDi), defined as the percentage change in arterial diameters between hyperemia and rest conditions: FMDi $= 100 \times (d_h - d_0)/d_0$. The physiological ability of relaxation of the endothelial vasculature can be assessed by administration of a 'NO donor' like GTN, which elicits a direct relaxation effect on the white muscular cells of the vessels. We evaluated the endothelium-independent vasodilation by a single dose (400 μg) of sublingual GTN. The brachial artery diameter was measured again 5 min after the spray administration (d_{gtn}). The endothelium-independent vasodilation was assessed by: GTNDi (percentage of dilation after GTN administration) $= 100 \times (d_{gtn} - d_0)/d_0$. The means (SD) of FMDi were 5.7% (6.2) in ICAD, 5.0% (9.3) in VAD, and 13.2% (6.5) in controls ($p < 0.0005$), without any difference between ICAD and VAD; mean values (SD) for endothelium-independent dilation were 21.5% (9.5) in patients with ICAD, 25.1% (12.5) in patients with VAD, and 20.8% (8.4) in controls, without significant difference

Table 2. Means (SD) of brachial artery diameter at rest (d_0), during hyperemia (d_h), and after glyceryl trinitrate (GTN) administration (d_{GTN}) in patients with cervical dissection of the internal carotid (ICAD) and vertebral (VAD) arteries, and in control subjects

	ICAD	VAD	Controls	p
Mean d_0 (SD) (mm)	3.95 (0.84)	3.82 (0.95)	3.99 (0.90)	0.73
Mean d_h (SD) (mm)	4.15 (0.75)	3.96 (0.87)	4.52 (1.03)	0.11
Mean d_{GTN} (SD) (mm)	4.76 (0.83)	4.69 (0.90)	4.79 (0.96)	0.89
Mean GTNDi (SD) (%)	21.5 (9.5)	25.1 (12.5)	20.8 (8.4)	0.49
Mean FMDi (SD) (%)	5.7 (6.2)*	5.0 (9.3)*	13.2 (6.5)	<0.0005

GTNDi = Percentage of dilation after GTN administration relative to the diameter at rest; FMDi = flow-mediated dilation index.

*Significant difference vs. controls.

between groups ($p = 0.49$). The brachial artery diameter at rest, after hyperemia, and after GTN administration did not differ between the three groups. Mean values (SD) for FMDi was 13.8% (6.5) in controls, 5.7% (6.2) in cases with ICAD, and 5.7% (8.9) in cases with VAD (table 2). The ANOVA on the ranks of FMDi with two factors: group of subjects with three levels (ICAD, VAD, and controls) and delay with two levels (before and after 783 days, median value), showed a significant effect of the group of subjects [$F(82.2) = 15.3$; $p < 0.001$], no effect of delay [$F(82.1) = 2.78$; $p = 0.78$], and no interaction. Post hoc analysis, using the Bonferroni correction for multiple comparisons, showed a significantly higher FMDi in controls than in patients with ICAD ($p = 0.002$) and VAD ($p < 0.001$), but no significant difference in FMDi between ICAD and VAD patients ($p = 0.28$). The ANOVA on GTNDi with the same factors did not show any significant effect of the group ($p = 0.49$). There were no differences between patients and controls for blood pressure, homocysteine, and total cholesterol levels and also for ex-smokers between groups.

Our study was the first to describe a significant impairment of endothelium-dependent vasodilation in patients with spontaneous CAD. This impairment is reflected by a decrease in the physiological response to an increase in blood flow. This occurs while vascular dilatory capabilities are preserved as demonstrated by a normal endothelium-independent vasodilation. The impairment of endothelium-dependent vasodilation is not just an acute phenomenon due to stroke, because patients were tested more than 80 days after stroke.

A significant difference in the FMDi between CAD patients and controls was observed. The endothelium-dependent vasodilation can thus be regarded as impaired in CAD patients, this happens irrespective of the location of the dissection, although ICAD and VAD patients are clinically considered as two different subtypes. The range of values obtained in CAD patients is similar to that reported in patients with endothelial dysfunction, whatever the etiology.

The vascular endothelium normally releases NO, a powerful relaxing factor, in response to many chemical and mechanical stimuli. One important stimulus of endothelial cell for NO release is the shear stress induced by the mechanical effects of blood flow [21]. The endothelium cell is sensitive to many vascular aggressive factors and its response to shear stress has been shown to be impaired in vascular diseases from their early stages. In spontaneous CAD, the pre-existence of an underlying tissue disorder has been often evoked. Connective tissue disorders like Marfan's syndrome [23] and polycystic kidney disease [24] have also been associated with CAD. Although these syndromes are rare, a minor form of extracellular matrix defect might be present in CAD patients. Recently, Wilson et al. [23] have reported a selective impairment of endothelium-dependent vasodilation in subjects with Marfan's syndrome. They have proposed a model explaining the relationship between endothelial dysfunction and cytoskeletal abnormalities of the arterial wall, and suggested a modified mechano-transduction of shear stress to NO release. This model might be applied to CAD patients and might explain the observed decrease in FMD.

Conclusion

Endothelium-dependent vasodilation is significantly impaired in subjects with spontaneous CAD, whereas endothelium-independent vasodilation is preserved. This finding strongly argues in favor of underlying ultrastructural abnormalities of the intima–media layers, predisposing to spontaneous CAD in some individuals. Further studies are needed to explain the relationship between endothelial function and cytoskeletal abnormalities of the arterial wall.

References

1 Fisher CM, Ojemann RG, Roberson GH: Spontaneous dissection of cervico-cerebral arteries. Can J Neurol Sci 1978;5:9–19.

2 Hart RG, Easton JD: Dissections of cervical and cerebral arteries. Neurol Clin 1983;1:155–182.

3 Leys D, Lesoin F, Pruvo JP, Gozet G, Jomin M, Petit H: Bilateral spontaneous dissection of extracranial vertebral arteries. J Neurol 1987;234:237–240.

4 Josien E: Extracranial vertebral artery dissection: Nine cases. J Neurol 1992;239:327–330.

5 Amarenco P, Seux-Levieil ML, Cohen A, Levy C, Touboul PJ, Bousser MG: Carotid artery dissection with renal infarcts. Two cases. Stroke 1994;25:2488–2491.

6 Tzourio C, Cohen A, Lamisse N, Biousse V, Bousser MG: Aortic root dilatation in patients with spontaneous cervical artery dissection. Circulation 1997;95:2351–2353.

7 Guillon B, Tzourio C, Biousse V, Adrai V, Bousser MG, Touboul PJ: Arterial wall properties in carotid artery dissection: An ultrasound study. Neurology 2000;55:663–666.
8 Furchgott RF, Zawadzki JV: The obligatory role of endothelial cells in the relaxation of arterial smooth muscle by acetylcholine. Nature 1980;288:373–376.
9 Vanhoutte PM, Rubanyi GM, Miller VM, Houston DS: Modulation of vascular smooth muscle contraction by the endothelium. Annu Rev Physiol 1986;48:307–320.
10 Rubanyi GM, Romero JC, Vanhoutte PM: Flow-induced release of endothelium-derived relaxing factor. Am J Physiol 1986;250:H1145–H1149.
11 Palmer RM, Ferrige AG, Moncada S: Nitric oxide release accounts for the biological activity of endothelium-derived relaxing factor. Nature 1987;327:524–526.
12 Pohl U, Herlan K, Huang A, Bassenge E: EDRF-mediated shear-induced dilation opposes myogenic vasoconstriction in small rabbit arteries. Am J Physiol 1991;261:H2016–H2023.
13 Celermajer DS, Sorensen KE, Gooch VM, Spiegelhalter DJ, Miller OI, Sullivan ID, Lloyd JK, Deanfield JE: Non-invasive detection of endothelial dysfunction in children and adults at risk of atherosclerosis. Lancet 1992;340:1111–1115.
14 Celermajer DS, Adams MR, Clarkson P, Robinson J, McCredie R, Donald A, Deanfield JE: Passive smoking and impaired endothelium-dependent arterial dilatation in healthy young adults. N Engl J Med 1996;334:150–154.
15 Panza JA, Quyyumi AA, Brush JE Jr, Epstein SE: Abnormal endothelium-dependent vascular relaxation in patients with essential hypertension. N Engl J Med 1990;323:22–27.
16 Chowienczyk PJ, Watts GF, Cockcroft JR, Ritter JM: Impaired endothelium-dependent vasodilation of forearm resistance vessels in hypercholesterolaemia. Lancet 1992;340:1430–1432.
17 Celermajer DS, Sorensen KE, Georgakopoulos D, Bull C, Thomas O, Robinson J, et al: Cigarette smoking is associated with dose-related and potentially reversible impairment of endothelium-dependent dilation in healthy young adults. Circulation 1993;88:2149–2155.
18 Lucas C, Lecroart JL, Gautier C, Leclerc X, Dauzat M, Leys D, Deklunder G: Impairment of endothelial function in patients with spontaneous cervical artery dissection: Evidence for a general arterial wall disease. Cerebrovasc Dis 2004;17:170–174.
19 Sorensen KE, Celermajer DS, Spiegelhalter DJ, Georgakopoulos D, Robinson J, Thomas O, Deanfield JE: Non-invasive measurement of human endothelium dependent arterial responses: Accuracy and reproducibility. Br Heart J 1995;74:247–253.
20 Leeson P, Thorne S, Donald A, Mullen M, Clarkson P, Deanfield J: Non-invasive measurement of endothelial function: Effect on brachial artery dilatation of graded endothelial dependent and independent stimuli. Heart 1997;78:22–27.
21 Adams MR, Robinson J, Sorensen KE, Deanfield JE, Celermajer DS: Normal ranges for brachial artery flow-mediated dilatation: A non-invasive ultrasound test of arterial endothelial function. J Vasc Invest 1996;2:146–150.
22 Goodfellow J, Ramsey MW, Luddington LA, Jones CJ, Coates PA, Dunstan F, Lewis MJ, Owens DR, Henderson AH: Endothelium and inelastic arteries: An early marker of vascular dysfunction in non-insulin dependent diabetes. Br Med J 1996;312:744–745.
23 Wilson DG, Bellamy MF, Ramsey MW, Goodfellow J, Brownlee M, Davies S, Wilson JF, Lewis MJ, Stuart AG: Endothelial function in Marfan syndrome: Selective impairment of flow-mediated vasodilation. Circulation 1999;99:909–915.
24 Leier CV, Baker PB, Kilman JW, Wooley CF: Cardiovascular abnormalities associated with adult polycystic kidney disease. Ann Intern Med 1984;100:683–688.

Christian Lucas, MD
Clinique Neurologique, Service de Neurologie Vasculaire
Hôpital Roger Salengro, CHRU de Lille
FR–59037 Lille Cedex (France)
Tel. +33 320 44 68 14, Fax +33 320 44 60 28, E-Mail clucas@chru-lille.fr

Baumgartner RW, Bogousslavsky J, Caso V, Paciaroni M (eds): Handbook on Cerebral Artery Dissection. Front Neurol Neurosci. Basel, Karger, 2005, vol 20, pp 70–76

Clinical Manifestations of Carotid Dissection

Ralf W. Baumgartner[a], *Julien Bogousslavsky*[b]

[a]Neurologische Klinik, Universitätsspital Zürich, Zürich, and
[b]Department of Neurology, Centre Hospitalier Universitaire Vaudois, Lausanne, Switzerland

Abstract

Spontaneous dissection of the cervical internal carotid artery (sICAD) causes, in more than 90% of patients, carotid territory ischemia, local signs and symptoms on the side of dissection, or both, whereas the remaining sICAD remain clinically asymptomatic. Local signs and symptoms include head, facial, or neck pain, Horner syndrome, pulsatile tinnitus, and cranial nerve palsy. Head, facial, or neck pain occurs in 64–74% and is the presenting symptom in up to 58.5%, and the only manifestation in 2.2–4.5%. Headache is observed in 65–68%, facial pain in 34–53%, and neck pain in 9–26%. Horner syndrome consisting essentially of miosis and ptosis is detected in 28–41%. Cranial nerve palsy is reported in 8–16%; the lower cranial nerves IX–XII are most commonly affected, in particular the hypoglossal nerve. The facial nerve may also be involved; dysgeusia results mainly from involvement of the chorda tympani (0.5–7.0%) or the glossopharyngeal nerve. Transient pareses of the ocular motor (III, IV and VI) and trigeminal nerves have been observed. Pulsatile tinnitus is reported in 16–27%. About three quarters of sICAD cause ischemic events, which include ischemic stroke in 80–84%, transient ischemic attack in 15–16%, amaurosis fugax in 3%, ischemic optic neuropathy in 4%, and retinal infarct in 1%. Patients with sICAD causing ischemia show a lower prevalence of Horner syndrome and palsy of the caudal cranial nerves than patients with sICAD causing no ischemic events, whereas headache, neck pain, and pulsatile tinnitus are equally frequent in both groups. After an ischemic stroke, independency defined by a moderate Rankin scale score of 0–2 occurs in 63–90%, whereas the outcome of retinal infarct and ischemic optic neuropathy are not well known.

Spontaneous dissection of the cervical internal carotid artery (sICAD) causes, in more than 90% of patients, ischemia in its territory, local signs and symptoms on the side of dissection, or both, while the remaining sICAD remain clinically asymptomatic [1]. Local signs and symptoms include head, facial, or neck pain, Horner syndrome, pulsatile tinnitus, and cranial nerve palsy [1–7]. Most symptomatic sICAD are accidentally detected during diagnostic work-up of patients with symptomatic dissection of the carotid or vertebral arteries [1].

Local Signs and Symptoms

Head pain (headache, facial, or neck pain) occurs in 64–74% of patients with sICAD. It is the presenting symptom of sICAD in up to 58.5% [1, 8], and the only manifestation in 2.2–4.5%. It is probable that the real prevalence of sICAD causing head pain only is higher, because not all patients with new acute headache undergo a screening for this disease. Furthermore, sICAD may imitate the symptom of a usual migraine attack [8], and such patients are unlikely to undergo the diagnostic work-up for sICAD. Intensity of pain is severe in 75% and mild to moderate in 25% [8]. Pain resolves in most patients, whereas persistent pain may suggest the presence of a dissecting aneurysm [7–9]. Head pain is assumed to be due to distension of the carotid wall by the dissection hematoma, which stimulates intramural pain-sensitive receptors.

Headache occurs in 65–68% of patients with sICAD and is typically unilateral, whereas bilateral headache occurs in 8–21% [1, 7, 8]. It is the presenting symptom in about half of patients, and other clinical symptoms develop after a median delay of 2.5 h (range 1–96 h) [7]. Headache involves generally the fronto-temporal area, but may affect the entire hemicranium or just the parieto-occipital area [7]. The onset of headache is usually gradual, but the patients may also describe 'thunderclap' headache [7]. The quality of the headache is perceived as aching in 66%, throbbing in 25%, and sharp in 7% [7]. The character of the headache is described as constant in 73% and pulsating in 25%, and 62% of patients consider it to be different from previously perceived headaches. On the other hand, about one fourth of patients with a history of migraine deem the headache to resemble their usual migraine attack [7, 8]. Headache lasts from 90 min to 30 days [8], and is resolved in 90% within 1 week [7].

Carotid dissection may rarely mimic cluster headache [10–12]. Oculosympathetic paralysis (ptosis and miosis) may also occur in the headache-free interval of primary cluster headache, whereas facial and supraorbital anhidrosis has not been observed, to our best knowledge, in this disease. sICAD may cause Horner syndrome, including essentially ptosis and miosis, while supraorbital anhidrosis is frequently absent. Thus, it may be difficult to differentiate primary from secondary disease forms in patients presenting with the first attacks of cluster headache.

Facial pain occurs in 34–53% of patients [7, 8]. The pain remains isolated in 7% of patients, and lasts from 2 h to 15 days [7, 8].

Neck pain is reported in 9–26% of patients, and is usually located in the upper anterolateral cervical region [1, 7, 8]. Pain lasts from 2 h to 15 days [8].

Although Horner syndrome consisting essentially of miosis and ptosis is as a well-known typical manifestation of sICAD, it is observed only in 28–41% of patients affected by this disease [1, 7, 8]. Supraorbital anhidrosis may also occur, because the supraorbital sweat glands are innervated by the internal carotid plexus [13]. Conversely, facial anhidrosis is typically absent, because the facial sweat glands are innervated by the sympathetic plexus surrounding the external carotid artery [13, 14]. A Horner syndrome is the only sign of sICAD in 10–12% [8, 14]. A recent multicenter observational study found a 12% stroke risk within 30 days after the onset of Horner syndrome in 90 patients with sICAD who presented with Horner syndrome with or without associated head pain, but no further neurological sign or symptom [15]. This observation suggests that an acute Horner syndrome should be considered as a medical emergency, and we recommend the urgent initiation of antithrombotic therapy in order to prevent ischemic stroke.

Cluster headache may mimic sICAD (see above). Fibromuscular dysplasia and/or dissection of the terminal (C1) internal carotid artery (ICA) causing striato-capsular infarct extending into the hypothalamus may imitate the symptoms of an sICAD, which causes headache, Horner syndrome, and contralateral hemiparesis [submitted]. Central Horner syndrome with contralateral hemiparesis may also result from thalamic infarct extending into the hypothalamus [16].

Cranial nerve palsy is reported in 8–16% of patients with sICAD [1, 3]. The lower cranial nerves IX–XII are most commonly affected, particularly the hypoglossal nerve, and the involvement of various combinations of nerves has been described [1, 3, 7]. Mechanical compression or stretching of the nerves by the expanded or aneurysmal ICA is the most likely explanation [1]. Transient tongue paralysis may occur after simultaneous central (brain infarct) and peripheral (dissection hematoma) lesion of the hypoglossal nerve [17]. The facial nerve may also be involved [1, 3], and facial diplegia was reported in a patient with bilateral sICAD [18]. Dysgeusia due to paresis of the chorda tympani has been observed in 0.5–7.0%, and it may occur without other cranial nerve involvement [1, 7, 19]. One patient suffering from dysgeusia due to palsy of the glossopharyngeal nerve without involvement of other cranial nerves has been reported [20]. The combination of the dysfunction of lower cranial nerves and Horner syndrome may be ascribed erroneously to a brain stem lesion.

In a few patients transient pareses of the ocular motor (III, IV and VI) and trigeminal nerves have been observed [3, 21, 22]. In case of sICAD not extending intracranially, the presumed cause is interruption of the nutrient arteries supplying the cranial nerves by hemodynamic, embolic, or both mechanisms

[21]. In case of sICAD extending into the cavernous sinus, mechanical compression or stretching of the cranial nerve is an alternative explanation [22].

Pulsatile tinnitus is reported in 16–27%, and an objective bruit may be present on auscultation [1, 7, 14, 23]. Tinnitus probably results from turbulences in the narrowed cervical ICA. A precise medical history may detect the transition from stenosis to occlusion as well as the subsequent recanalization of sICAD by the disappearance and transient reappearance of a pulsatile tinnitus, respectively.

Carotid Territory Ischemia

About three quarters of sICAD cause ischemic events, which include ischemic stroke in 80–84%, transient ischemic attack in 15–16%, amaurosis fugax in 3%, ischemic optic neuropathy in 3.6%, and retinal infarct in 1% [1, 24, 25]. All ischemic events in 144 patients with 145 symptomatic sICAD consisted of ischemic stroke in 80%, transient ischemic attack in 39%, amaurosis fugax in 18%, and retinal infarct in 5% [unpubl. observations]. Earlier studies reported a higher prevalence of carotid territory ischemia, probably because nowadays the condition is diagnosed in more patients with less obvious manifestations [2, 7].

sICAD causing carotid territory ischemia show a lower prevalence of Horner syndrome ($p < 0.001$) and palsy of the caudal cranial nerves ($p < 0.01$) than sICAD causing no ischemic events [1]. Headache, neck pain, and pulsatile tinnitus are equally frequent in both groups [1]. Furthermore, sICAD causing carotid territory ischemia show more, often severe, stenoses and occlusions of the cervical ICA ($p < 0.0001$) and obstructions of the middle or anterior cerebral arteries ($p < 0.001$), and a trend for more associated vascular risk factors that is significant for hypercholesterolemia ($p < 0.05$) compared to sICAD causing no ischemia.

Retinal and Optic Nerve Ischemia. As mentioned above, transient retinal ischemia seems to be a frequent symptom of sICAD, whereas retinal infarct, anterior and posterior ischemic optic neuropathy are rare manifestation of this disease [1–3, 6, 9, 24–30]. Whereas retinal ischemia results from arterio-arterial embolism, optic nerve ischemia is assumed to be due to a hemodynamic failure [24]. The outcome of blindness related to retinal and optic nerve ischemia is not well known. In 3 of 4 patients with ischemic optic neuropathy one patient regained normal visual acuity, whereas visual field deficit persisted in the second patient, and blindness persisted in the other 2 patients [24].

Ischemic Stroke. Only about one fifth of patients suffer an ischemic stroke without any warning signs [2]. The clinical signs and symptoms correspond to those observed in territorial infarcts of the middle cerebral artery. The reason is that the overwhelming majority of patients suffer embolic middle cerebral artery territory strokes, and infarcts in the territory of the anterior and posterior cerebral arteries as well as watershed infarcts are rare [31–33].

The clinical outcome of patients with ischemic stroke due to sICAD is not well known. Series of patients with space-occupying ('malignant') middle cerebral artery infarct have reported that the cause of stroke is sICAD in 11–30% [34–38]. The main reason for this high number of sICAD patients is probably selection bias, because younger patients such as those with sICAD are more likely to be referred to a center with a stroke unit [39]. One-month outcome was investigated in a recent study examining 73 patients with ischemic stroke due to mainly sICAD causing carotid occlusion [33]. The patients were derived from a population-based primary care center, and underwent conservative therapy, as no hemicraniectomy, hypothermia, or thrombolysis was performed. After one month, 63% of cases had a modified Rankin scale score of 0–2, 20% of 3–5, and 17% were dead [33]. Conversely, series with less sICAD cases reported excellent or good recovery from ischemic stroke in 70–90% [40–42]. The low numbers of investigated patients and differences in patient selection are the most probable explanation of the different clinical outcomes.

References

1 Baumgartner RW, Arnold M, Baumgartner I, Mosso M, Gönner F, Studer A, Schroth G, Schuknecht B, Sturzenegger M: Carotid dissection with and without ischemic events: Local symptoms and cerebral artery findings. Neurology 2001;57:827–832.

2 Biousse V, D'Anglejan-Chatillon J, Massiou H, Bousser MG: Time course of symptoms in extracranial carotid artery dissections. A series of 80 patients. Stroke 1995;26:235–239.

3 Mokri B, Silbert PL, Schievink WI, Piepgras DG: Cranial nerve palsy in spontaneous dissection of the extracranial internal carotid artery. Neurology 1996;46:356–359.

4 Schievink W, Mokri B, Garrity JA, Nichols DA, Piepgras DG: Ocular motor nerve palsies in spontaneous dissections of the cervical internal carotid artery. Neurology 1993;43:1938–1941.

5 Schievink WI, Mokri B, O'Fallon WM: Recurrent spontaneous cervical artery dissection. N Engl J Med 1994;330:393–397.

6 Schievink WI: Spontaneous dissection of the carotid and vertebral arteries. N Engl J Med 2001; 344:899–906.

7 Silbert PL, Mokri B, Schievink WI: Headache and neck pain in spontaneous internal carotid and vertebral artery dissections. Neurology 1995;45:1517–1522.

8 Biousse V, D'Anglejan-Chatillon J, Massiou H, Bousser MG: Head pain in non-traumatic carotid artery dissection: A series of 65 patients. Cephalalgia 1994;14:33–36.

9 Mokri B, Sundt TMJ, Houser OW, Piepgras DW: Spontaneous dissection of the cervical internal carotid artery. Ann Neurol 1986;19:126–138.

10 Frigerio S, Bühler R, Hess CW, Sturzenegger M: Symptomatic cluster headache in internal carotid artery dissection – Consider anhidrosis. Headache 2003;43:896–900.

11 Lance JW: Migrainous neuralgia or cluster headache. J Neurol Sci 1971;13:401–414.

12 Rosebraugh CJ, Griebel DJ, DiPette DJ: A case report of carotid dissection presenting as cluster headache. Am J Med 1997;102:418–419.

13 Watson C, Vijayan N: The sympathetic innervation of the eyes and face: a clinicoanatomic review. Clin Anat 1995;8:262–272.
14 Hart RG, Easton JD: Dissection of cervical and cerebral arteries. Neurol Clin 1983;1:155–182.
15 de Bray J-M, Baumgartner RW, Guillon B, Pautot V, Dziewas R, Ringelstein EB, Sturzenegger M, Garniers P, Ducrocq X, Saudeau S, Neau J-P, Larrue V, Vuilllier F, Bouillat J, Verret J-M, Verny C, Dubas F: Isolated Horner's syndrome may herald stroke. Cerebrovasc Dis 2005;19:274–275.
16 Rossetti AO, Reichhart MD, Bogousslavsky J: Central Horner's syndrome with contralateral ataxic hemiparesis: A diencephalic alternate syndrome. Neurology 2003;61:334–338.
17 Mouradian MS, Chan KM, Jeerakathil T, Shuaib A: Transient total tongue paralysis from simultaneous central and peripheral lesions. J Neurol Neurosurg Psychiatry 2001;70:806–808.
18 Gout O, Bonnaud I, Weill A, Moulignier A, Quenet JJ, Moret J, Bakouche P: Facial diplegia complicating a bilateral internal carotid artery dissection. Stroke 1999;30:681–686.
19 Schievink WI: A surgeon with a nasty taste in his mouth. Lancet 1997;350:260.
20 Taillibert S, Bazin B, Pierrot-Deseilligny C: Dysgeusia resulting from internal carotid dissection. A limited glossopharyngeal nerve palsy. J Neurol Neurosurg Psychiatry 1998;64:691–692.
21 Schievink WI, Mokri B, Garrity JA, Nichols DA, Piepgras DG: Ocular motor nerve palsies in spontaneous dissections of the cervical internal carotid artery. Neurology 1993;43:1938–1941.
22 Maitland CG, Black JL, Smith WA: Abducens nerve palsy due to spontaneous dissection of the internal carotid artery. Arch Neurol 1983;40:448–449.
23 Fisher CM, Ojemann RG, Robertson GH: Spontaneous dissection of the cervico-cerebral arteries. Can J Neurol Sci 1978;5:9–19.
24 Biousse V, Schaison M, Touboul P-J, D'Anglejan-Chatillon J, Bousser MG: Ischemic optic neuropathy associated with internal carotid artery dissection. Arch Neurol 1998;55:715–719.
25 Touzé E, Gauvrit JY, Moulin T, Meder JF, Bracard S, Mas JL, for the Multicenter Survey on Natural History of Cervical Artery Dissection. Risk of stroke and recurrent dissection after a cervical artery dissection. A multicenter study. Neurology 2003;61:1347–1351.
26 Biousse V, Touboul PJ, D'Anglejan-Chatillon J, Levy C, Schaison M, Bousser MG: Ophthalmologic manifestations of internal carotid artery dissection. Am J Ophthalmol 1998; 126:565–577.
27 Bogousslavsky J, Despland PA, Regli F: Spontaneous carotid dissection with acute stroke. Arch Neurol 1987;44:137–140.
28 McNeill DH, Dreisbach J, Marsden RJ: Spontaneous dissection of the internal carotid artery: its conservative management with heparin sodium. Arch Neurol 1980;37:54–55.
29 Newman NJ, Kline LB, Leifer D, Lessell S: Ocular stroke and carotid artery dissection. Neurology 1989;39:1462–1464.
30 Rivkin MJ, Hedges TR, Logigian EL: Carotid dissection as posterior ischemic optic neuropathy. Neurology 1990;40:1469.
31 Benninger DH, Georgiadis D, Kremer C, Studer A, Nedeltchev K, Baumgartner RW: Mechanism of ischemic infarct in spontaneous carotid dissection. Stroke 2004;35:482–485.
32 Lucas C, Moulin T, Deplanque D, Tatu L, Chavot D, the DONALD Investigators: Stroke patterns of internal carotid artery dissection in 40 patients. Stroke 1998;29:2646–2648.
33 Milhaud D, de Freitas GR, van Melle G, Bogousslavsky J: Occlusion due to carotid artery dissection: A more severe disease than previously suggested. Arch Neurol 2002;59:557–561.
34 Berrouschot J, Sterker M, Bettin S, Köster J, Schneider D: Mortality of space-occupying ('malignant') middle cerebral artery infarction under conservative intensive care. Intensive Care Med 1998;24:620–623.
35 Georgiadis D, Schwarz S, Aschoff A, Schwab S: Hemicraniectomy and moderate hypothermia in patients with severe ischemic stroke. Stroke 2002;33:1584–1588.
36 Heinsius T, Bogousslavsky J, Van Melle G: Large infarcts in the middle cerebral artery territory. Etiology and outcome patterns. Neurology 1998;50:341–350.
37 Schwab S, Steiner T, Aschoff A, Schwarz S, Steiner HH, Jansen O, Hacke W: Early hemicraniectomy in patients with complete middle cerebral artery infarction. Stroke 1998;29:1888–1893.
38 Walz B, Zimmermann C, Bottger S, Haberl RL: Prognosis of patients after hemicraniectomy in malignant middle cerebral artery infarction. J Neurol 2002;249:1183–1190.

39 Nedeltchev K, Auf der Maur T, Georgiadis D, Arnold M, Caso V, Mattle HP, Schroth G, Remonda L, Sturzenegger M, Fischer U, Baumgartner RW: Ischemic stroke in young adults: Predictors of outcome and recurrence. J Neurol Neurosurg Psychiatry 2005;76:2191–2195.
40 Engelter ST, Lyrer PA, Kirsch EC, Steck AJ: Long-term follow-up after extracranial internal carotid artery dissection. Eur Neurol 2000;44:199–204.
41 Leys D, Moulin T, Stoijkovic T, Begey S, Chavot D: Follow-up of patients with history of cervical artery dissection. Cerebrovasc Dis 1995;5:43–49.
42 Sturzenegger M: Spontaneous internal carotid artery dissection. Early diagnosis and management in 44 patients. J Neurol 1995;242:231–238.

Ralf W. Baumgartner, MD
Department of Neurology, University Hospital
Frauenklinikstrasse 26, CH–8091 Zürich (Switzerland)
Tel. +41 1 255 56 86, Fax +41 1 255 88 64
E-Mail ralf.baumgartner@usz.ch

Baumgartner RW, Bogousslavsky J, Caso V, Paciaroni M (eds): Handbook on Cerebral Artery Dissection. Front Neurol Neurosci. Basel, Karger, 2005, vol 20, pp 77–86

Clinical Manifestations of Vertebral Artery Dissection

Marcel Arnold[a], *Marie-Germaine Bousser*[b]

[a]Department of Neurology, University Hospital of Bern, Bern, Switzerland;
[b]Department of Neurology, University Hospital Lariboisière, Paris, France

Abstract

The most frequent clinical manifestation of vertebral artery dissection is posterior headache or neck pain accompanied or followed by posterior circulation transient ischemic attack or stroke. Rarer clinical features include isolated headache or neck pain, cervical spinal cord ischemia and cervical root impairment. Asymptomatic vertebral artery dissections have been reported.

In the case of primary intracranial vertebral artery dissection or intracranial extension of an extracranial dissection, subarachnoid hemorrhage and rarely rostral cervical spinal cord ischemia or posterior fossa mass effect may occur.

Vertebral artery dissection (VAD) is a potentially disabling and yet probably under-recognised condition often occurring in young and middle-aged adults. The mean age of symptom onset is about 40 years. But VAD can occur also in children and in patients older than 60 years [1, 2]. The classical clinical presentation is occipital headache, posterior neck pain, or both, usually more marked on the side of the dissection associated with posterior circulation ischemia (table 1). There is often a time delay of some hours or days between the occurrence of pain and ischemia.

However, the spectrum of clinical presentation is broad. Some patients present with headache or neck pain alone and asymptomatic patients with proven VAD have been described. If the dissection extends intracranially subarachnoid hemorrhage (SAH) or lower brain stem compression may occur. All clinical symptoms and signs are not specific for VAD. Therefore the diagnosis

Table 1. Clinical findings in patients with extracranial vertebral artery dissection

Occipital headache and/or posterior neck pain
History of neck or head trauma
Posterior circulation TIA (e.g. vertigo, vomiting, diplopia, visual blurring, dysphagia, gait disturbance, facial numbness, motor symptoms)
Posterior circulation stroke (often lateral medullary syndrome)
Cervical spinal cord ischemia (middle cervical segments, rare)
Cervical root impairment (mostly at the C5–C6 level, rare)

of VAD is more difficult than the diagnosis of carotid artery dissection, where often a painful Horner syndrome or lower cranial nerve palsies accompanied by pain are helpful in establishing the diagnosis.

VAD may occur spontaneously without any triggering events, but it is also observed after preceding infection, mostly of the respiratory tract [3], during pregnancy or after delivery [4], or after a major or minor neck or head trauma. There are clearly dissections of traumatic origin following serious head or neck trauma such as motor vehicle accident and penetrating trauma. However, the relation of trauma and VAD is a complex issue and the role of trivial trauma, daily activities, and sport activities, such as minor falls, intubation, sneezing, coughing, ceiling painting, forced head turning, tennis, roller-coaster [5], yoga, and skiing, in the pathogenesis of dissections is not clear and a reliable differentiation between spontaneous and traumatic dissection is not possible.

An association between chiropractic manipulation and VAD has been described. In adults younger than 45 years, vertebral dissection patients were five times more likely than healthy controls to have been treated by a chiropractor within one week prior to the dissection [6]. Cervical manipulation may precipitate a stroke in patients with cervical pain as the only symptom of VAD [7].

A history of migraine is more frequent in patients with cervical artery dissection compared with healthy controls [8].

In more than 10% of patients multivessel cervical artery dissections occur simultaneously [9–11]. Data about multiple simultaneous dissections are scarce. Therefore it remains unclear, whether these patients represent a group with other predisposing intrinsic factors or precipitating events leading to a transient arteriopathy.

In recent years VAD has been diagnosed more frequently since new imaging techniques allow early and reliable diagnosis. Nevertheless the knowledge about clinical manifestations of VAD is based on small case series and case reports.

Extracranial Vertebral Artery Dissection

Headache and/or Neck Pain

Occipital headache or posterior neck pain or both are a prominent and early finding in most patients [1]. In a series of Sturzenegger [12] 12 of 14 patients complained of pain preceding ischemia. The pain was predominantly unilateral and ipsilateral to the dissected artery, but was also reported to be bilateral. Pain was usually sudden, sharp, severe, and different from previous pain episodes.

Silbert et al. [1] described 26 patients with VAD. Twenty-three percent of them had a history of migraine. In 69% headache was a presenting symptom of VAD, mostly ipsilateral to the dissected artery, in 83% of the patients with headache it was located posteriorly, but rare cases of frontal or generalized headache were observed. The predominantly occipital location of headache may be explained by the innervation of this region by the upper cervical nerves. Headache had a pulsatile character in 44% and was steady in 56%. The pain tended to be more pulsatile in character in patients with a history of migraine. In the majority of patients (72%) onset of pain was gradual; however, about a fourth of the patients complained of abrupt onset of pain. In single cases a sudden exacerbation after an initial gradual onset may occur. Only 50% of the patients described their headache as unique. Pain preceded other clinical manifestations in many patients. The mean time interval from pain to ischemia onset was 3.7 days (median 14.5 h; range 1 h to 14 days). The mean duration of headache associated with VAD was 8.3 days (median 3 days, range 2–35 days). None of the 26 patients developed chronic headache or aggravation of pre-existing migraine or tension-type headaches after the dissection.

In the same series neck pain was observed in 46% of the patients, more than half of them with accompanying headache. Neck pain developed usually gradually and was unilateral in two thirds and bilateral in one third of the patients. It radiated to the shoulder in only one patient. Neck pain was the initial clinical symptom in 5 patients with a time interval between neck pain to other symptoms of 12 days (median 14 days, range 0.5–30 days). Delays of more than one month between VAD and ischemic stroke are rare and have been reported only in single cases [13].

In a Canadian series of 26 patients with 32 VAD, headache and/or neck pain occurred in 88% of the patients, in 53% as a warning symptom preceding posterior circulation ischemia [14].

Pain may be unilateral even in the case of bilateral dissection [15].

In VAD patients, pain may be transient, absent, or of minor intensity. Therefore, musculoskeletal neck pain is often difficult to distinguish from the pain of vertebral dissection, although in patients with dissection physical examination does not usually reveal any muscle tenderness or restriction of neck mobility. Even in vertebral dissection patients with severe neck pain, clinical examination of the neck, and the entire neurological examination may be unremarkable [12]. The situation is more complex in patients with traumatic dissection in whom pain and tenderness of neck muscles may be due to the musculoskeletal trauma. Cervical manipulation in such patients may aggravate the situation dramatically with upward extension of the dissection, and sometimes lethal brain stem infarction [7]. We thus recommend avoidance of all cervical manipulations, and imaging of the brain and cervical magnetic resonance imaging (MRI) with T1 fat-suppression techniques in patients with unusual occipital headache or neck pain, especially in association with symptoms of posterior circulation ischemia.

Posterior Circulation Ischemia

More than 80% of patients develop posterior circulation ischemia [1, 16]. Transient ischemic attacks (TIA) or stroke may occur by embolism from the dissected artery or by hemodynamic impairment of the territory supplied by an occluded or severely stenosed vertebral artery.

Lateral medullary infarction (Wallenberg syndrome or partial Wallenberg syndrome) is common, consisting of ipsilateral Horner syndrome, sensory disturbances on the ipsilateral face, nystagmus, ipsilateral limb ataxia, and contralateral impairment of pain and thermal sensation. The patient typically complains about vertigo, nausea, vomiting, dysphagia, hoarseness, ataxia, and facial numbness. Other clinical manifestations include cerebellar, thalamic, pontine, and posterior cerebral artery infarcts [15]. Medial medullary syndromes (ipsilateral hypoglossal nerve paresis and contralateral hemiparesis) associated with VAD have been described [17]. In the case of basilar artery occlusion due to embolism from the dissected artery or extension of the dissection to the basilar artery, severe brainstem stroke causing locked-in syndrome or death may occur. A patient who experienced a transient 'locked-in' state has been described [18].

In a Canadian series of 26 patients with VAD, the main clinical symptoms included vertigo in 57%, cerebellar signs in 33%, and lateral medullary signs in 26% [14].

Another series reported 9 completed strokes in 13 patients with VAD [11]. Only 2 of these strokes were preceded by TIA. The prevalence of lateral medullary syndrome was 30% in this study.

In an unpublished study of 92 consecutive patients of the university hospitals of Bern and Zürich [own unpubl. data], the main clinical symptom was stroke in 75 patients (81.5%), TIA in 10 (10.9%), SAH in 1 (1.1%), and isolated headache and/or neck pain in 4 (4.4%). In 2 patients with simultaneous carotid artery dissection, VAD was asymptomatic. The median National Institute of Health Stroke Scale score on admission was 4 (range 0–35). The interval from symptom onset to diagnosis ranged from 2h to 31 days (median interval, 2 days). The majority of our VAD patients (83%) presented with posterior neck pain, or occipital headache, or both as in other series [1, 10]. In spite of these typical clinical presentations diagnosis was delayed in many patients with a time interval from symptom onset to diagnosis of up to 31 days (median 2 days). These findings strike the need for further improvement of patient and doctor awareness for VAD because the symptoms and signs of VAD are not familiar to many emergency physicians and most of the patients.

An important differential diagnosis is migraine. Migraine attacks may present with posterior headache although entire hemicrania is typical. Photophobia and phonophobia, nausea, and vomiting may be present in migraine patients. However, symptoms of cerebellar or brainstem ischemia may be similar to the so-called basilar migraine symptoms. Therefore in any migraine patient with a headache attack recognized by the patient as different from his usual attacks immediate MRI/magnetic resonance angiography of the cervical arteries with a standard dissection protocol should be performed.

Spinal Cord Ischemia

The intracranial vertebral arteries supply branches to the rostral cervical spinal cord segments. The middle cervical spinal segments are perfused by anterior and posterior radicular branches of the extradural vertebral artery at several levels. Therefore, embolic or hemodynamic infarction of the cervical spinal cord may occur as an unusual complication of VAD [19]. In a recent report 7 patients with spinal cord ischemia due to VAD were reviewed [20]. Ischemia was in the territory of the posterior spinal artery in 3 patients, and of the anterior spinal artery territory in 2 patients. Two patients presented with combined cervical spinal cord and medullary ischemia. Unilateral infarctions were associated with ipsilateral VAD. Bilateral infarction was found in 2 patients with unilateral and in one patient with bilateral VAD. Anterior and posterior radicular arteries may arise predominantly or only from one vertebral artery. This explains why bilateral spinal cord infarction may occur in unilateral VAD.

Cervical Root Impairment

Radicular syndromes caused by VAD have been very rarely described. Proximal paresis of an arm due to cervical root impairment most commonly occurs at the C5–C6 level [20]. In a recent review of 6 patients, pain and weakness were more prominent than sensory deficits and 5 patients had a minor trauma preceding the dissection [20].

Cervical roots may be compressed or stretched by arterial enlargement by a subadventitial mural hematoma or a dissecting aneurysm. Another explanation may be ischemia of the nutrient artery to the spinal root originating from the anterior or posterior radicular arteries.

The clinician has to be aware that VAD leading to cervical root impairment is a rare differential diagnosis in patients with a painful cervical radicular syndrome without compression by disc material or osteophytes and without signs of infectious or neoplastic radicular disease.

Asymptomatic Patients

Some patients with VAD may be asymptomatic even without headache, with the VAD being detected during the diagnostic procedures in patients with symptoms and signs of carotid dissection [10]. In a patient with acoustic neurinoma VAD, as an incidental finding, was reported [21]. In an asymptomatic patient with migraine and Marfan syndrome, a VAD was observed by chance at the time of repeat angiography after previous carotid artery dissection [22].

Intracranial Vertebral Artery Dissection

Intracranial dissection may occur purely intracranially or due to the upward extension of an extracranial VAD to the ipsilateral intracranial segment of the vertebral artery. In a recent French series of 42 patients with extracranial VAD, 38% of the patients had an ipsilateral intradural extension of the dissection [23]. The clinical presentation of intracranial VAD can include both posterior circulation ischemia and SAH, mostly associated with posterior headache or neck pain [24]. Posterior fossa mass effect is another rare manifestation [25]. The various clinical manifestations of intracranial VAD are summarized in table 2. Because of the risk of both ischemia and SAH, the treatment of intracranial VAD is particularly difficult.

Table 2. Clinical findings in patients with intracranial vertebral artery dissection

Generalized or occipital headache and/or posterior neck pain
History of neck or head trauma
Subarachnoid hemorrhage
Posterior circulation ischemia TIA (e.g. vertigo, vomiting, diplopia, visual blurring, dysphagia, gait disturbance, facial numbness, motor symptoms)
Posterior circulation stroke (often lateral medullary syndrome)
Posterior fossa syndrome with lower cranial nerve compression (rare)
Cervical spinal cord ischemia (rostral cervical segment, rare)
Spinal subarachnoid hemorrhage (rare)

Headache and/or Neck Pain

Intracranial VAD occurs spontaneously in most cases, and presents often with posterior headache or neck pain. In a Japanese series of 31 patients headache, posterior neck pain, or both were present in 55% of the patients [24]. Intensity of posterior headache or neck pain was severe in the majority of cases. However, 5 patients complained only about mild headache or neck dullness. Pain location was holocranial or frontal in some patients, and posterior head or neck pain was bilateral in more than half of the patients. In another small study headache was sometimes occipital but more often generalized and preceded the onset of ischemia in some patients by many days [25]. Another study reported 2 of 6 patients with intracranial VAD without any headache or neck pain and emphasized the need of imaging the vertebral artery by MRI/magnetic resonance angiography in the clinical setting of young patients with posterior circulation ischemia [26].

Posterior Circulation Ischemia

Intracranial VAD often leads to a unilateral brainstem syndrome including lateral medullary syndrome [25]. In some of these patients infarcts may progress and lead to coma and tetraparesis. Multiple posterior circulation strokes may occur. The patients with infarction following intracranial VAD had an average age of 39 years [25].

In a Japanese series of 31 patients with intracranial VAD, 15 had posterior circulation infarction, 7 of them Wallenberg syndrome, 5 other brain stem infarction, one cerebellar infarction and 2 cerebral infarction, 4 patients had vertebrobasilar TIAs, one sudden deafness, one headache only, 4 an asymptomatic aneurysm, 3 an asymptomatic dissection without aneurysm, and 3 patients a SAH [24]. The mean age of the patients was 55 years (range 25–82 years). The most frequent initial clinical symptoms were severe headache, vertigo, nausea, and vomiting. Other less frequent symptoms included dysarthria, tinnitus, double vision, dysesthesia, consciousness disturbance, hemiparesis, and dysphasia. In 9 of these 31 patients, a possibly precipitating trauma associated with the dissection was identified.

Subarachnoid Hemorrhage

SAH occurs when the dissection is subadventitial and tears the adventitia. The vessel walls of intracranial cerebral arteries are thinner than those of extracranial cerebral arteries. This may explain that rupture through the thin adventitia with extravascular bleeding of the intracranial vertebral artery may occur. SAH has been reported in 1 of 10 patients with intracranial VAD [15]. In a recent French study 2 of 16 patients with an intracranial extension of an extracranial VAD suffered an SAH [23].

Patients with SAH had an average age of 49 years and present often with prodromal headache or with moderate to severe sudden onset of headache [25]. Neck pain may be prominent but the severity and location of pain was not different from aneurysmal bleeding in patients with other causes than dissection. More than half of the patients had previous hypertension.

In a Japanese series of 24 patients with SAH due to intracranial VAD, on admission 9 patients had a grade I or II on the Hunt and Kosnik scale, and 15 patients a Hunt and Konsnik grade III, IV, or V. Severe neurological deficits on admission, re-bleeding episode(s) and lesions with a pearl-and-string structure were predictive of poor outcome.

Single cases of spinal SAH associated with VAD have been described [20]. The patient presented with acute chest pain radiating to the back and neck and rapidly progressive myelopathy.

In any case of unexplained SAH the clinician has to consider intracranial VAD as a potential cause. However, it may be difficult to distinguish a stenosis caused by VAD and a spasm due to the SAH on angiography. Therefore, MRI is needed to confirm the diagnosis.

Posterior Fossa Mass Effect

Posterior fossa mass effect with compression of lower brain stem and cranial nerves caused by a dissecting aneurysm of the vertebral artery without bleeding were rarely reported [25, 27, 28].

Conclusions

The clinical features of VAD are broad and vary from asymptomatic patients to severe lethal brain stem stroke. The typical clinical presentation is headache or neck pain followed or accompanied by posterior circulation ischemia. Less common clinical manifestations include isolated headache or neck pain, cervical root impairment and cervical spinal cord ischemia. In patients with intracranial VAD, posterior circulation ischemia, SAH, and rarely rostral cervical spinal cord ischemia or posterior fossa mass effect may be present.

The diagnosis of VAD may be difficult when only local symptoms are present. Neck pain and headache are frequently located posteriorly. However, the pain of VAD does not often have a unique and worrying character. Therefore VAD pain is frequently misinterpreted as musculoskeletal neck pain or tension headache and the true incidence of VAD is very likely to be much higher than reported. VAD may have devastating consequences, which can often be avoided when early diagnosis is made. This implies that the patient presenting with any unexplained headache or neck pain should be investigated for VAD by adequate imaging.

Extracranial VAD may extend to the intracranial segment of the vertebral artery and the basilar artery. Therefore SAH should be ruled out by appropriate investigations before anticoagulants are administered.

References

1 Silbert PL, Mokri B, Schievink WI: Headache and neck pain in spontaneous internal carotid and vertebral artery dissections. Neurology 1995;45:1517–1522.

2 Schievink WI, Mokri B, Piepgras DG: Spontaneous dissections of cervicocephalic arteries in childhood and adolescence. Neurology 1994;44:1607–1612.

3 Guillon B, Berthet K, Benslamia L, Bertrand M, Bousser MG, Tzourio C: Infection and the risk of spontaneous cervical artery dissection: A case-control study. Stroke 2003;34:79–81.

4 Mas JL, Bousser MG, Corone P, Touboul PJ: Aneurysme dissequant des arteres vertebrales et grossesse. Rev Neurol 1987;11:761–764.

5 Biousse V, Chabriat H, Amarenco P, Bousser MG: Roller-coaster induced vertebral artery dissection. Lancet 1995;346:767.

6 Rothwell DM, Bondy SJ, Williams JI: Chiropractic manipulation and stroke: A population-based case-control study. Stroke 2001;32:1054–1060.

7 Mas JL, Henin D, Bousser MG, Chain F, Hanno JJ: Dissecting aneurysm of the vertebral artery and cervical manipulation. A case report with autopsy. Neurology 1989;39:512–515.

8 Tzourio C, Benslamia L, Guillon B, Aidi S, Bertrand M, Berthet K, Bousser MG: Migraine and the risk of cervical artery dissection: A case-control study. Neurology 2002;59:435–437.

9 Mas JL, Goeau C, Bousser MG, Chiras J, Verret JM, Touboul PJ: Spontaneous dissecting aneurysms of the internal carotid and vertebral arteries – Two case reports. Stroke 1985;16: 125–129.

10 Schievink WI, Mokri B, O'Fallon WM: Recurrent spontaneous cervical-artery dissection. N Engl J Med 1994;330:393–397.

11 Mas JL, Bousser MG, Hasboun D, Laplane D: Extracranial vertebral artery dissection: A review of 13 cases. Stroke 1987;18:1037–1047.
12 Sturzenegger M: Headache and neck pain: The warning symptoms of vertebral artery dissections. Headache 1995;34:187–193.
13 Nazir FS, Muir KW: Prolonged interval between vertebral artery dissection and ischemic stroke. Neurology 2004;62:1646–1647.
14 Saeed AB, Shuaib A, Al-Sulaiti G, Emery D: Vertebral artery dissection: Warning symptoms, clinical features and prognosis in 26 patients. Can J Neurol Sci 2000;27:292–296.
15 Mokri B, Houser OW, Sandok BA, Piepgras DG: Spontaneous dissection of the vertebral arteries. Neurology 1988;38:880–885.
16 Schievink WI: Spontaneous dissection of the carotid and vertebral arteries. N Engl J Med 2001;344:899–906.
17 Leppert D, Radue EW: Medial medullary syndrome due to vertebral artery dissection. J Neurol Neurosurg Psychiatry 2001;70:130–131.
18 Hicks PA, Leavitt JA, Mokri B: Ophthalmic manifestations of vertebral artery dissection. Ophthalmology 1994;101:1786–1792.
19 Leys D, Lucas G, Gobert M, Deklunder G, Pruvo JP: Cervical artery dissections. Eur Neurol 1997;37:3–12.
20 Crum B, Mokri B, Fulgham J: Spinal manifestations of vertebral artery dissection. Neurology 2000;55:304–306.
21 Mascalchi M, Bianchi MC, Mangiafico S, Ferrito G, Puglioli M, Marin E, Mugnai S, Canapicchi R, Quilici N, Inzitari D: MRI and MR angiography of vertebral artery dissection. Neuroradiology 1997;39:329–340.
22 Youl BD, Coutellier A, Dubois B, Leger JM, Bousser MG: Three cases of spontaneous extracranial vertebral artery dissection. Stroke 1990;21:618–625.
23 Garnier P, Demasles S, Januel AC, Michel D: Intracranial extension of extracranial vertebral artery dissections. A review of 16 cases. Rev Neurol (Paris) 2004;160:679–684.
24 Hosoya T, Adachi M, Yamaguchi K, Haku T, Kayama T, Kato T: Clinical and neuroradiological features of intracranial vertebrobasilar artery dissection. Stroke 1999;30:1083–1090.
25 Caplan LR, Baquis GD, Pessin MS, D'Alton J, Adelman LS, DeWitt LD, Ho K, Izukawa D, Kwan ES: Dissection of the intracranial vertebral artery. Neurology 1988;38:868–877.
26 Provenzale JM, Morgenlander JC, Gress D: Spontaneous vertebral dissection: Clinical, conventional angiographic, CT, and MR findings. J Comput Assist Tomogr 1996;20:185–193.
27 De Busscher J: Anéurysme de l'artère vertébrale gauche chez un home 45 ans. Acta Neurol Psychiatr Belg 1952;52:1–23.
28 Miyazaki S, Yamaura A, Kamata K, Fukushima H: A dissecting aneurysm of the vertebral artery. Surg Neurol 1984;21:171–174.

Marcel Arnold, MD
Department of Neurology, University Hospital of Bern
Inselspital
CH–3010 Bern (Switzerland)
Tel. +41 31 632 33 32, Fax +41 31 632 96 79, E-Mail marcel.arnold@insel.ch

Baumgartner RW, Bogousslavsky J, Caso V, Paciaroni M (eds): Handbook on Cerebral Artery Dissection. Front Neurol Neurosci. Basel, Karger, 2005, vol 20, pp 87–101

Ultrasound Assessment of Cervical Artery Dissection

D.H. Benninger[a], *V. Caso*[b], *R.W. Baumgartner*[a]

[a]Department of Neurology, University Hospital, Zürich, Switzerland;
[b]Stroke Unit, Division of Internal and Cardiovascular Medicine, University of Perugia, Perugia, Italy

Abstract

The purpose of this chapter is to present ultrasound and, in particular, color duplex sonography (CDS) assessment of spontaneous dissection of the cervical internal carotid (sICAD) and vertebral (sVAD) arteries. The examination, typical ultrasound findings and pitfalls in the acute sICAD and sVAD, detection of microembolic signals, and recanalization will be discussed.

Examination

The examination of the anterior cerebral circulation (fig. 1) includes extracranially the insonation of (1) the common carotid artery (CCA), (2) the external carotid artery, (3) the origin and (4) the cervical part of the internal carotid artery (ICA). The orbital window is used to assess the carotid siphon and the ophthalmic arteries (OphA). Transtemporal insonation with an axial plane depicts the precommunicating (A1) anterior cerebral artery and mainly in case of cross-flow the anterior communicating arteries, the sphenoidal (M1) and insular (M2) segments of the middle cerebral artery (MCA), and somewhat caudally, the cervical segment (C1) of the ICA [1]. In the posterior part of the temporal window, the pre- (P1) and postcommunicating (P2) posterior cerebral and the posterior communicating arteries are visualized [1–3]. By tilting the ultrasound transducer 10° upwards, parts of the postcommunicating (A2) anterior cerebral artery, M2 and opercular (M3) MCA are identified [1, 2]. The additional use of the coronal plane is useful for unequivocal differentiation of

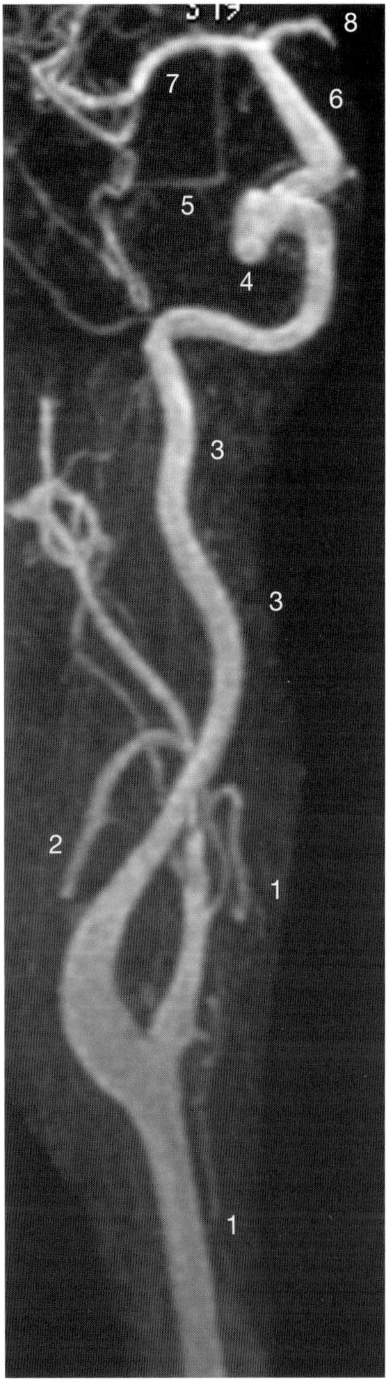

Fig. 1. Cerebral artery insonation for assessing spontaneous dissection of the internal carotid artery (1 = common carotid artery; 2–5 = different segments of the internal carotid artery: 2 = origin; 3 = cervical segment; 4 = horizontal segment of the petrosal part; 5 = carotid siphon; 6 = terminal (C1) segment; 7 = middle cerebral artery; 8 = anterior and anterior communicating arteries).

the basal cerebral arteries [4]. The anterior coronal plane shows A1 anterior cerebral artery, M1 MCA, and C1 ICA, whereas the posterior coronal plane visualizes P1 and P2 posterior cerebral artery, the posterior communicating artery, M2 and M3 MCA, and sometimes the tip of the basilar artery (BA) [4]. We routinely insonate also the horizontal segment of the pars petrosa of the ICA using axial and coronal planes [5], because spontaneous ICA dissection may rarely cause flow velocity increase in this part of the ICA, whereas the cervical ICA still has normal flow velocities. Furthermore, the hemodynamic findings observed in the pars petrosa may be helpful to distinguish sICAD causing subtotal stenosis from those leading to occlusion.

The right CCA, most parts of the left CCA, the origin and proximal parts of the ICA, and the external carotid artery can be assessed with high-frequency (4–8 MHz) linear transducers. Thus, the wall of the aforementioned cerebral arteries can be depicted with B-mode imaging in most patients. Due to the increasing distance between the insonated vessel and the ultrasound probe, the examination of the proximal part of the left CCA and distal parts of the cervical ICA, and transorbital and -temporal studies are performed with low-frequency (1.8–3.6 MHz) sector (or Doppler) probes, which have a significantly lower resolution at B-mode and color Doppler imaging than linear probes. Furthermore, a precondition for successful transtemporal insonation is the use of low-frequency ultrasound probes. With respect to sICAD, the proximal parts of the cervical ICA can be investigated with linear transducers, which enable spectral and color Doppler sonography as well as B-mode imaging. Conversely, distal parts of the cervical ICA must be insonated with sector (or Doppler) transducers, which allow mainly the detection of hemodynamic abnormalities, whereas the carotid wall cannot be examined.

The investigation of the posterior cerebral circulation consists extracranially of the insonation of the subclavian artery, and the origin (V0), the prevertebral part (V1), the pars transversaria (V2), and the atlas loop (V3) of the vertebral (VA) artery. Transnuchal (transforaminal) insonation allows the unequivocal identification of both VA and V3 from the intracranial (V4) segment. Both VA stick together at insonation depths of 70–71 mm and form the BA [6, 7]. The BA can often be followed up to the top, located at insonation depths of up to 110 mm. The additional use of the sagittal planes may prove useful, when the VA and BA are not clearly identified in the axial plane.

The V0, V1, and V2 segments of the right VA, the V1, and V2 segments of the left VA, the right subclavian artery, and most parts of the left subclavian artery, with the exception of the origin can be assessed with linear transducers. The investigation of the atlas loop (V3) may be difficult with linear transducers. Conversely, the origin and proximal part of the left CCA, the left V0 and V1, both V4 and the BA must be insonated with sector (or Doppler) probes. SVAD

Table 1. Presenting color duplex ultrasound findings in 181 patients with 200 spontaneous carotid dissections with and without ischemic events

	Ischemia (n = 145) n (%)	No ischemia (n = 55) n (%)	All (n = 200) n (%)
Atherosclerotic carotid artery plaque	13 (9)	2 (4)	15 (8)
Cervical ICA-vessel wall thickened and hypoechogenic	36 (25)	12 (22)	48 (24)
Second lumen	3 (2)	1 (2)	4 (2)
Dissecting aneurysm	1/10 (10)[1]	0/7 (0)[2]	1/17 (6)[3]
Normal hemodynamics	7 (5)**	16 (29)**	24 (12)
Stenosis			
≤50%	7 (5)*	9 (16)*	16 (8)
51–80%	10 (7)	8 (15)	18 (9)
>80% or occlusion	120 (83)**	22 (40)**	142 (71)
Intracranial stenosis or occlusion[4]	43 (30)	2 (4)	45 (23)
Median latency (range) symptom onset – ultrasonography	2 (0–90) days	10 (0–125) days	10 (0–125) days

ICA = Internal carotid artery.

[1]10 of 101 dissections showed an aneurysm at catheter or MR angiography; [2]7 of 44 dissections showed an aneurysm at catheter or MR angiography; [3]17 of 145 dissections showed an aneurysm at catheter or MR angiography; [4]middle and anterior cerebral arteries.

$^{*}p < 0.01$, $^{**}p < 0.0001$ that the difference between carotid dissections with and without ischemia is significant (Wilcoxon signed-rank test).

can affect all segments of the VA [8–13]. Thus, the right V0, V1, V2 (and often V3) can be investigated with linear transducers, which allow the detection of vessel wall abnormalities. Conversely, the remaining VA segments must be investigated with sector (or Doppler) transducers, which enable essentially the identification of hemodynamic abnormalities, while wall abnormalities are hardly depicted.

Ultrasound Findings in Acute sICAD

The prerequisite for ultrasound diagnosis of acute sICAD is the presence of no or at best mild atherosclerosis in the cerebral arteries [14–22]. Typical B-mode and color Doppler imaging findings may be observed in acute sICAD, but they are not validated by 'gold standards' like MR imaging and angiography. Thus, diagnosis of sICAD is mainly based on the detection of abnormal

Table 2. Color duplex ultrasound findings in 135 patients with 142 spontaneous carotid dissections

Cervical internal carotid artery	
Stenosis	
Intrastenotic flow velocity	
Increased	14 (10)
Decreased	51 (36)
Occlusion	77 (54)
Cross-flow through	
Anterior communicating artery	111 (78)
Posterior communicating artery	75 (53)
Anterior and/or posterior communicating arteries	136 (96)
Ophthalmic artery	72 (51)

Values are numbers, with percentages in parentheses.

hemodynamic findings (stenosis or occlusion) in the cervical ICA. Presenting color duplex sonography (CDS) findings observed in 181 own patients with 200 sICAD are summarized in tables 1 and 2.

The sensitivity of combined extracranial Doppler and duplex sonography and transcranial Doppler sonography (TCD) for diagnosis of sICAD is 95–100% [16, 21–23]. The sensitivity of extra- and transcranial CDS for detecting 145 sICAD causing carotid territory ischemia was 95%, and for detecting 55 sICAD causing no ischemic event 71% [15]. No study has investigated the specificity, positive, and negative predictive values of ultrasound assessment of sICAD.

B-Mode and Color Doppler Imaging Findings in Acute sICAD

B-mode and color Doppler imaging findings observed in the cervical ICA of patients with sICAD include luminal narrowing, thickened and hypoechogenic vessel wall, intimal flap, and pseudoaneurysm.

Compared to atherosclerotic carotid stenosis, *luminal narrowing* in sICAD begins a few centimeters after the origin of the ICA and extends over a longer distance (fig. 2; unpubl. data).

Mural hematoma and intraluminal thrombus may be detected as *thickened and hypoechogenic vessel wall* [16, 18]. As already mentioned, the dissection hematoma typically begins a few centimeters after the origin of the ICA or may even be located a few centimeters below the base of the skull. The cervical ICA has a length of about 8 cm, and mainly the proximal part of the vessel wall can be investigated with linear scans providing an appropriate resolution. The aforementioned anatomical and physical facts are the main reason, why an

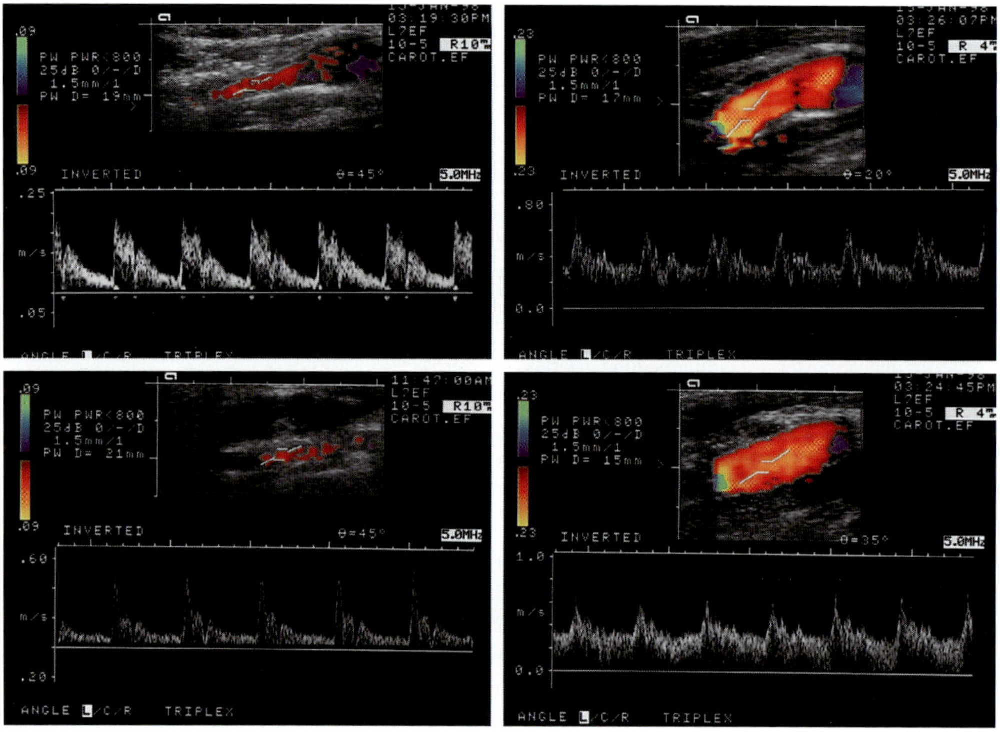

a *b* *c* *d*

Fig. 2. Extracranial color duplex sonography shows on the left side (***a***, ***c***) the findings at the origin (***a***) and in the mid-cervical portion (***c***) of a spontaneously dissected internal carotid artery, and on the right side (***b***, ***d***) the corresponding findings at the origin (***b***) and the mid-cervical portion (***d***) of the opposite normal internal carotid artery. The dissected carotid artery shows pathologically slow flow velocities affecting especially the diastolic component and a reduced luminal diameter compared to the normal vessel.

abnormal vessel wall was just detected in about 25% of 200 own sICAD (unpubl. data). Although wall hematoma and intraluminal thrombus cannot be reliably differentiated by B-mode imaging, the identification of intraluminal blood flow and the intima reflex allows the reliable detection of the wall hematoma, sometimes [16, 18, 20, 21, 24] (fig. 3).

An *intimal flap* is defined as a flat hyperechogenic structure bordering the presumed intramural hematoma, floating in the lumen or separating two lumina with different Doppler signals [16, 19–24]. It is important to note that intimal flaps must be distinguished from the wall of the adjacent jugular vein. In our experience, intimal flaps are a rare finding in sICAD (table 1).

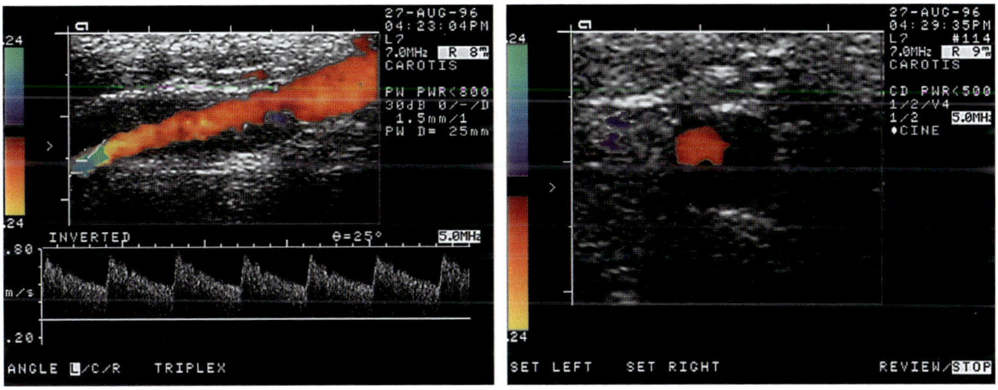

a *b*

Fig. 3. Extracranial color duplex sonography of a spontaneously dissected internal carotid artery shows at longitudinal (***a***) and (***b***) axial planes the thickened vessel wall resulting from a hypoechogenic mural hematoma, whereas the flow velocities are normal.

CDS visualized one of 17 (6%) *pseudoaneurysms* which were found at catheter and MR angiographies performed in acute sICAD (unpubl. data) [15]. The reason for the low detection rate is most likely the fact that the aneurysms are located in the depth of the neck and must thus be investigated with low-frequency transducers. Furthermore, it is difficult to reliably distinguish ICA redundancies from aneurysmal dilatation.

It is difficult to identify the *intimal laceration* leading to intramural bleeding and dissection of the carotid wall at histological examination of autopsy and endarterectomy specimens [25, 26]. Thus, it is unlikely that ultrasound may reliably depict an intimal tear in patients with sICAD.

Hemodynamic Findings in Acute sICAD

Abnormal hemodynamics in the cervical ICA of patients with acute sICAD has been consistently found in ultrasound studies, severe stenosis and occlusion being the most frequent findings [15–17, 19, 21, 22]. Considering the dynamic nature of sICAD with complete recanalization even within days [21], the time interval between the onset of symptoms and the ultrasound study influences the number of abnormal findings in the cervical ICA [15].

Criteria for diagnosis of different degrees of stenosis and occlusion in sICAD have been published recently [15]. A *≤50% stenosis of the cervical ICA* is diagnosed in the presence of increased intrastenotic peak systolic velocity (PSV) (women, >90 cm/s; men, >80 cm/s) and a PSV quotient intrastenotic ICA/contralateral cervical ICA >1.12; each reference value is higher than the PSV mean value plus three standard deviations of own healthy volunteers.

A *51–80% stenosis of the cervical ICA* is diagnosed in the presence of an intrastenotic PSV >120 cm/s and a PSV quotient intrastenotic ICA/CCA on the side of sICAD (ipsilateral) >1.5. *Severe (>80%) stenoses of the cervical ICA* caused decreased intrastenotic flow velocities in 78% of 65 sICAD (fig. 2), and focally increased intrastenotic flow velocities in the remaining cases (table 2; unpubl. data), which is an accordance with the results of previous studies [17]. Therefore, severe stenoses are diagnosed using pre- and poststenotic hemodynamic criteria, and at least two of the following three have to be present: (1) the quotient of the resistance index (RI, PSV – peak diastolic velocity/PSV) of ipsilateral CCA/RI of contralateral CCA is >0.15; (2) reversal of flow in the ipsilateral OphA, and (3) cross-flow through the anterior communicating arteries. The criteria for 51–80 and 81–99% ICA stenoses have been published in peer-reviewed journals, developed in studies using catheter angiography as standard of reference, and elaborated with the same ultrasound equipment as is used in the laboratory of the present authors [27–29]. The last criterion is important, because different ultrasound machines have been shown to measure different flow velocities under identical conditions of examination in both flow phantoms and patients [30]. *Occlusion of the cervical ICA* was assessed as reported before [22]. Using catheter angiography as standard of reference, it has been shown that ultrasound may misdiagnose subtotal stenosis as occlusion in acute ICAD [22]. Therefore, some authors group acute sICAD causing >80% stenosis and occlusion together [15].

Pitfalls of Ultrasound Diagnosis of sICAD

As mentioned before, diagnosis of sICAD is mainly based on the detection of stenosis, which may cause increased or decreased intrastenotic flow velocities, or occlusion in the cervical ICA. Conditions, which are associated with no or mild atherosclerosis and cause (1) increased flow velocities in the cervical ICA, (2) decreased flow velocities in the cervical ICA, or (3) an occlusion of the cervical ICA may thus mimic sICAD, and are discussed below.

(1) Conditions associated with increased flow velocities in the cervical ICA may result either from a stenosis or from increased blood flow and flow velocity. Redundancies of the cervical ICA, such as kinking, coiling, and looping, may mimic ≤50% stenosis, and it is impossible to differentiate whether raised flow velocity in a redundant artery results from the redundancy itself or an additional stenosis. Furthermore, carotid redundancies seem to be more prevalent in patients with sICAD [31, 32]. Fibromuscular dysplasia may also cause a stenosis of the cervical ICA. Although ultrasound may detect the irregular stenoses and aneurysmal dilatations ('string of beads') associated with fibromuscular dysplasia [33–36], most cases are missed. Vasospasm is a rare cause of transient cervical ICA stenosis [37]. The absence of signs of sICAD at cervical magnetic

resonance imaging (MRI) and catheter angiography, and spasm resolution with time point to the diagnosis. Increased blood flow and flow velocities (and sometimes also vessel diameter) in the cervical ICA may be observed in large (diameter >4mm) arteriovenous malformations of the brain [38] and carotid cavernous fistulas [39, 40]. Another cause of increased flow and flow velocities in the ICA is a persistent primitive trigeminal artery, which connects the intracranial ICA with the BA. The additional presence of hypoplastic VA and direct visualization of the persistent primitive vessel by transcranial CDS may allow the suspicion of the diagnosis, which must be confirmed by magnetic resonance angiography. Increased blood flow, flow velocities, and heart rate may be observed in medical diseases such as anemia and hyperthyreosis. The presence of increased flow velocities in all cerebral arteries and the identification of the corresponding clinical and laboratory findings will allow the diagnosis.

(2) Conditions associated with decreased flow velocities in the cervical ICA include severe stenosis or occlusion of the intracranial ICA or MCA. Patients with occlusion of the lower carotid siphon show reduced flow velocities without diastolic component in the cervical ICA, and reversed flow in the homolateral OphA. Patients with severe intracranial carotid stenosis or occlusion located distal to the origin of the OphA, occlusion of the intracranial ICA, or M1 MCA occlusion often show decreased flow velocities in the ipsilateral cervical ICA. The antegrade flow direction in the OphA will point towards a severe stenosis or occlusion of the upper siphon or C1 ICA, but this sign is not always reliable. Nevertheless, it is literally impossible to decide in the abovementioned cases, whether the decreased flow velocities in the cervical ICA are due to the intracranial obstruction alone or the intracranial obstruction and an associated sICAD. This diagnostic problem arises in young adults with acute MCA territory stroke and occlusion of M1 MCA or C1 ICA.

(3) Conditions associated with an occlusion of the cervical ICA. As reported in the chapter by Paciaroni et al. (pp. 102–118), angiographic findings observed in acute sICAD causing an occlusion are nonspecific, and the same applies to the hemodynamic ultrasound findings. Intravascular thrombus may extend into the carotid bulb over time and the distinction from atherothrombotic occlusion may become difficult. We have observed 2 patients with potential cardiac source of embolism and occlusion of the cervical ICA, which recanalized completely within 3 months. Both aforementioned patients had no local signs, such as Horner syndrome, on the side of ICA obstruction, and no signs of ICAD at MR imaging of the neck and catheter angiography (unpubl. data).

Detection of Microembolic Signals by TCD in sICAD

TCD has been used to detect microembolic signals in the MCA supplied by a dissected cervical ICA [41–43]. Microembolic signals were more

Table 3. Color duplex ultrasound findings at presentation and one-year follow-up in 200 spontaneous carotid dissections[1]

	Presentation (n = 200) n (%)	Follow-up (n = 188) n (%)
Atherosclerotic carotid artery plaque	15 (8)	19 (10)
Cervical ICA-vessel wall thickened and hypoechogenic	48 (24)	0
Second lumen	4 (2)	0
Dissecting aneurysm	1/17 (6)	1/17 (6)
Normal	24 (12)	110 (59)
Stenosis		
≤50%	16 (8)	17 (9)
51–80%	18 (9)	3 (2)
81–99%	75 (38)	17 (9)
Occlusion	77 (34)	41 (22)
Intracranial stenosis or occlusion[2]	45 (23)	0

ICA = Internal carotid artery.

[1]200 dissections occurred in 181 patients; ultrasonic follow-up was obtained in 188 carotid dissections, because 3 dissections had caused lethal strokes, 3 dissections had no follow-up, and 6 dissections were excluded for other reasons (thrombolytic therapy for acute stroke, surgical, or endovascular therapy of the dissected carotid artery).

[2]Middle and anterior cerebral arteries.

frequently observed in patients with carotid territory ischemia than without [41, 43]. Preliminary data suggest that microembolic signals detection on serial TCD studies may be associated with an increased risk of early recurrence of ischemic events [42, 44].

Follow-Up Investigation in sICAD

Recanalization of the obstructed ICA results from the resorption of the mural hematoma and the intraluminal thrombus. Steinke et al. [21] used Doppler sonography to study the recanalization of 50 angiographically proven sICAD. Recanalization was observed in 34 vessels (68%) after an average time interval of 51 days [21]. Sturzenegger et al. [22] detected sICAD recanalization in 63% of 43 patients, whereas occlusion persisted in 37%. We found less favorable data in 188 sICAD examined one year after symptoms onset: complete recanalization was present in 59%, a ≤50% stenosis in 9%, a 51–80% stenosis in 2%, a 81–99% stenosis in 9%, and an occlusion in 22% (table 3; unpubl. data).

Ultrasound Findings in Acute sVAD

Ultrasound diagnosis of acute sVAD is based on the detection of abnormal B-mode and color Doppler imaging and hemodynamic findings. Pathological hemodynamic findings observed in patients with acute sVAD are nonspecific, and just their location in the V2 or V3 segments, which is rarely affected by other vascular disease, suggests that dissection might be the underlying cause. The sensitivity of pathological hemodynamics for diagnosis of sVAD has been validated in small monocenter series including up to 20 patients with 24 sVAD; MRI and angiography were used as standard of reference [8–10, 12, 13]. Sensitivity for detecting patients with *extracranial sVAD* was 75% in a study examining 20 cases with CDS [8], and 86% in 7 patients examined with extracranial CDS and continuous-wave Doppler and TCD [9]. The sensitivity for detecting patients with *extra- and intracranial sVAD* using was 86% in 14 patients insonated with extracranial pulsed-wave Doppler and duplex sonography and TCD [12]. The sensitivity for detecting intracranial sVAD was 100% in 9 patients examined with extracranial CDS and continuous-wave Doppler and TCD [9]. As in sICAD, no study has investigated the specificity, positive, and negative predictive values of ultrasound assessment of sVAD.

B-Mode and Color Doppler Imaging Findings in Acute sVAD

Imaging abnormalities detected in patients with sVAD include irregular stenosis, thickened and hypoechogenic vessel wall, dissecting membrane with true and false lumen, pseudoaneurysm, and tapering stenosis with distal occlusion [8, 10]. Touboul et al. [13] described the combination of local increase in vessel diameter with hemodynamic signs of stenosis or occlusion at the same level and decreased pulsatility and presence of intravascular echoes in the enlarged vessel as typical findings. A subsequent study using extracranial CDS and TCD observed the aforementioned sign in 2 of 11 (18%) extracranial sVAD.

Hemodynamic Findings in Acute sVAD

The hemodynamic criteria used for diagnosis of VA stenosis and occlusion in patients with sVAD and atherosclerotic VA disease are identical, although they vary somewhat between different authors [8–13, 45–48]. *VA stenosis* is defined by a focal increase of flow velocity, while a severe stenosis is associated with intrastenotic, bi-directional, low-frequency and high-intensity signals, as well as prestenotic (increased RI) and poststenotic (decreased RI) hemodynamic abnormalities [9]. However, a severe stenosis extending over several centimeters may also cause decreased intrastenotic flow velocities (unpubl. data). In *VA occlusion* there are neither intraluminal spectral and color Doppler signals nor wall motion during the heart cycle, and B-mode imaging may disclose intraluminal echoes resulting from the fresh thrombus [8–13, 45–48]. In *occlusion of proximal (V0 or V1) VA*, there are often cervical collaterals, which enter V2 or V3 and lead to undulating or antegrade flow in V4 [46, 48]. *Occlusion of V4 before the origin of the posterior inferior cerebellar artery* (PICA) is associated with abnormally slow systolic but no diastolic flow velocities, and often-reversed flow is detected in the distal V4, which irrigates the PICA [9, 45–47]. *Occlusion of V4 located after the origin of the PICA* is associated with slow systolic and slow but preserved diastolic flow velocities, whereas the distal V4 VA is not detected at transforaminal insonation [9, 45–47]. *Occlusion of V3* may lead to the same pre- and postocclusional hemodynamic findings as in occlusion of V4 before the origin of the PICA, or the whole V4 VA may show a high-resistance profile with no diastolic flow velocities and reversed flow direction (unpubl. data).

Pitfalls of Ultrasound Diagnosis of Acute sVAD

It may be difficult to differentiate V4 occlusion from VA hypoplasia. Hypoplastic VA shows slow systolic and diastolic flow velocities, may disclose undulating but not reversed flow in V4, and the connection with the VA will be absent in hypoplastic VA, which end in the PICA [49]. The differentiation from a V4 occlusion is feasible by detection of a small vessel diameter, the preserved diastolic velocities in preocclusional VA, and reversed flow in postocclusional VA in case of VA occlusion located before the origin of the PICA. However, the diagnosis of sVAD in a hypoplastic vessel is very difficult, especially when the occlusion is located after the origin of the PICA.

Follow-Up Investigation in sVAD

Recanalization of *extracranial* sVAD causing stenosis was found in 8 of 10 (80%) cases and in 2 of 7 (29%) occlusions after a mean follow-up of 8 months [8]. De Bray et al. [9] reported recanalization in 3 of 6 (50%) extracranial stenoses and 1 of 3 (33%) extracranial occlusions.

Recanalization of *intracranial* sVAD causing stenosis was observed in 6 of 11 (55%) cases and in 1 of 3 (33%) occlusions [9].

Conclusion

The high sensitivity of ultrasound for detecting acute sICAD in patients with carotid territory ischemia suggests that it may suffice to exclude this disease, in particular when the ultrasound study is performed by an experienced sonographer. The aforementioned pitfalls leading to falsely positive results advocate that ultrasound suspicion of acute sICAD must be confirmed by cervical MRI and magnetic resonance angiography. The lower sensitivity of ultrasound for assessing patients with acute sICAD causing no ischemic event and patients with acute sVAD indicate that those patients should principally undergo MRI of the neck and angiography. Ultrasound is useful for noninvasive monitoring of vessel recanalization and guiding the antithrombotic therapy.

References

1 Bogdahn U, Becker G, Winkler J, Greiner K, Perez J, Meurers B: Transcranial color-coded real-time sonography in adults. Stroke 1990;21:1680–1688.

2 Baumgartner RW, Baumgartner I, Mattle HP, Schroth G: Transcranial color-coded duplex sonography in the evaluation of collateral flow through the circle of Willis. AJNR Am J Neuroradiol 1997;18:127–133.

3 Klötzsch C, Popescu O, Berlit P: Assessment of the posterior communicating artery by transcranial color-coded duplex sonography. Stroke 1996;27:486–489.

4 Baumgartner RW, Mattle HP, Aaslid R, Kaps M: Transcranial color-coded duplex sonography in arterial cerebrovascular disease. Cerebrovasc Dis 1997;7:57–63.

5 Baumgartner RW, Mattle HP, Aaslid R: Transcranial color-coded duplex sonography, magnetic resonance angiography, and computed tomography angiography: Methods, applications, advantages, and limitations. J Clin Ultrasound 1995;23:89–111.

6 Kaps M, Seidel G, Bauer T, Behrmann B: Imaging of the intracranial vertebrobasilar system using color-coded ultrasound. Stroke 1992;23:1577–1582.

7 Schöning M, Walter J: Evaluation of the vertebrobasilar-posterior system by transcranial color duplex sonography in adults. Stroke 1992;23:1280–1286.

8 Bartels E, Flügel KA: Evaluation of extracranial vertebral artery dissection with duplex color-flow imaging. Stroke 1996;27:290–295.

9 de Bray JM, Penisson-Besnier I, Dubas F, Emile J: Extracranial and intracranial vertebrobasilar dissections: Diagnosis and prognosis. J Neurol Neurosurg Psychiatry 1997;63:46–51.

10 Lu CJ, Sun Y, Jeng JS, Huang KM, Hwang BS, Lin WH, Chen RC, Yip PK: Imaging in the diagnosis and follow-up evaluation of vertebral artery dissection. J Ultrasound Med 2000;19:263–270.

11 Röther J, Schwartz A, Rautenberg W, Hennerici M: Magnetic resonance angiography of spontaneous vertebral artery dissection suspected on Doppler ultrasonography. J Neurol 1995;242: 430–436.

12 Sturzenegger M, Mattle HP, Rivoir A, Rihs F, Schmid C: Ultrasound findings in extracranial vertebral artery dissection. Stroke 1993;24:1910–1921.

13 Touboul PJ, Mas JL, Bousser MG, Laplane D: Duplex scanning in extracranial vertebral artery dissection. Stroke 1987;18:116–121.

14 Houser OW, Mokri B, Sundt TMJ, Baker HL, Reese DF: Spontaneous cervical cephalic arterial dissection and its residuum: Angiographic spectrum. AJNR Am J Neuroradiol 1984;5:27–34.

15 Baumgartner RW, Arnold M, Baumgartner I, Mosso M, Gönner F, Studer A, Schroth G, Schuknecht B, Sturzenegger M: Carotid dissection with and without ischemic events: Local symptoms and cerebral artery findings. Neurology 2001;57:827–832.

16 de Bray JM, Lhoste P, Dubas F, Emile J, Saumet JL: Ultrasonic features of extracranial carotid dissections: 47 cases studied by angiography. J Ultrasound Med 1994;13:659–664.

17 Hennerici M, Steinke W, Rautenberg W: High resistance flow pattern in extracranial carotid artery dissection. Arch Neurol 1989;46:670–672.

18 Logason K, Hardemark HG, Barlin T, Bergqvist D, Ahlstom H, Karacagil S: Duplex scan findings in patients with spontaneous cervical artery dissections. Eur J Vasc Endovasc Surg 2002;23: 295–298.

19 Mullges W, Ringelstein EB, Leibold M: Non-invasive diagnosis of internal carotid artery dissections. J Neurol Neurosurg Psychiatry 1992;55:98–104.
20 Sidhu PS, Jonker ND, Khaw KT, Patel N, Blomley MJ, Chaudhuri KR, Frackowiak RS, Cosgrove DO: Spontaneous dissections of the internal carotid artery: Appearances on colour Doppler ultrasound. Br J Radiol 1997;70:50–57.
21 Steinke W, Rautenberg W, Schwartz A, Hennerici M: Noninvasive monitoring of internal carotid artery dissection. Stroke 1994;25:998–1005.
22 Sturzenegger M, Mattle HP, Rivoir A, Baumgartner RW: Ultrasound findings in carotid artery dissection: Analysis of 43 patients. Neurology 1995;45:691–698.
23 Treiman GS, Treiman RL, Foran RF, Levin PM, Cohen JL, Wagner WH, Cossmann DV: Spontaneous dissection of the internal carotid artery: A nineteen-year clinical experience. J Vasc Surg 1996;24:597–607.
24 Clevert DA, Rupp N, Reiser M, Jung EM: Improved diagnosis of vascular dissection by ultrasound B-flow: A comparison with color-coded Doppler and power Doppler sonography. Eur Radiol 2005;151:342–347.
25 de Bray JM, Baumgartner RW: History of carotid dissection. Arch Neurol 2005; in press.
26 Gauthier G, Rohr J, Wildi E, Megret M: L'hématome disséquant spontané de l'artère carotide interne. Revue générale de 205 cas publiés dont 10 personels. Schweiz Arch Neurol Psychiatr 1985;136:53–74.
27 Moneta G, Edwards JM, Chitwood RW, Taylor D, Lee RW, Cummings CA, Porter JM: Correlation of North American Symptomatic Carotid Endarterectomy Trial (NASCET) angiographic definition of 70% to 99% internal carotid artery stenosis with duplex scanning. J Vasc Surg 1993;17:152–159.
28 Polak JF, Dobkin GR, O'Leary DH, Wang AM, Cutler SS: Internal carotid artery stenosis: Accuracy and reproducibility of color-Doppler-assisted duplex imaging. Radiology 1989;173:793–800.
29 Whiters CE, Gosink BB, Keightley AM, Casola G, Lee AA, van Sonnenberg E, Rotrock JF, Lyden PD: Duplex carotid sonography. Peak systolic velocity in quantifying internal carotid artery stenosis. J Ultrasound Med 1990;9:345–349.
30 Fillinger MF, Baker RJ Jr, Zwolak RM, Musson A, Lenz JE, Mott J, Bech FR, Walsh DB, Cronenwett JL: Carotid duplex criteria for a 60% or greater angiographic stenosis: Variation according to equipment. J Vasc Surg 1996;24:856–864.
31 Barbour PJ, Castaldo JE, Rae-Grant AD, Gee W, Reed JF 3rd, Jenny D, Longennecker J: Internal carotid artery redundancy is significantly associated with dissection. Stroke 1994;25:1201–1206.
32 Ozdoba C, Sturzenegger M, Schroth G: Internal carotid artery dissection: MR imaging features and clinical-radiologic correlation. Radiology 1996;199:191–198.
33 Arning C, Grzyska U: Color Doppler imaging of cervicocephalic fibromuscular dysplasia. Cardiovasc Ultrasound 2004;20:1–7.
34 Edell SL, Huang P: Sonographic demonstration of fibromuscular hyperplasia of the cervical internal carotid artery. Stroke 1981;12:518–520.
35 Perren F, Urbano L, Rossetti AO, Ruchat P, Uske A, Meuli R, Lobrinus JA, Bogousslavsky J, Devuyst G: Ultrasound image of a single symptomatic carotid stenosis disclosed as fibromuscular dysplasia. Neurology 2004;62:1023–1024.
36 Winter R, Ringleb P, Hacke W: Color-coded duplex ultrasound imaging of intimal fibromuscular dysplasia of the carotid artery. Nervenarzt 1998;69:905–908.
37 Arning C, Schrattenholzer A, Lachenmayer L: Cervical carotid artery vasospasms causing cerebral ischemia. Detection by immediate vascular ultrasonographic investigation. Stroke 1998;29:1063–1066.
38 Baumgartner RW, Mattle HP, Schroth G: Transcranial color-coded duplex sonography of cerebral arteriovenous malformations. Neuroradiol 1996;38:734–737.
39 Chen YW, Jeng JS, Liu HM, Hwang BS, Lin WH, Yip PK: Carotid and transcranial color-coded duplex sonography in different types of carotid-cavernous fistula. Stroke 2000;31:701–706.
40 Lin HJ, Yip PK, Liu HM, Hwang BS, Chen RC: Noninvasive hemodynamic classification of carotid-cavernous sinus fistulas by duplex carotid sonography. J Ultrasound Med 1994;13:105–113.

41 Koennecke HC, Trocio SH Jr, Mast H, Mohr JP: Microemboli on transcranial Doppler in patients with spontaneous carotid artery dissection. J Neuroimaging 1997;7:217–220.

42 Molina CA, Alvarez-Sabin J, Schonewille W, Montaner J, Rovira A, Abilleira S, Codina A: Cerebral microembolism in acute spontaneous internal carotid artery dissection. Neurology 2000;55:1738–1740.

43 Srinivasan J, Newell DW, Sturzenegger M, Mayberg MR, Winn HR: Transcranial Doppler in the evaluation of internal carotid artery dissection. Stroke 1996;27:1226–1230.

44 Droste DW, Junker K, Stogbauer F, Lowens S, Besselmann M, Braun B, Ringelstein EB: Clinically silent circulating microemboli in 20 patients with carotid or vertebral artery dissection. Cerebrovasc Dis 2001;12:181–185.

45 Kimura K, Yasaka M, Moriyasu H, Tsuchiya T, Yamaguchi T: Ultrasonographic evaluation of vertebral artery to detect vertebrobasilar axis occlusion. Stroke 1994;25:1006–1009.

46 Ringelstein EB, Zeumer H, Poeck K: Non-invasive diagnosis of intracranial lesions in the vertebrobasilar system. A comparison of Doppler sonographic and angiographic findings. Stroke 1985;16:848–855.

47 Saito K, Kimura K, Nagatsuka K, Nagano K, Minematsu K, Ueno S, Naritomi H: Vertebral artery occlusion in duplex color-coded ultrasonography. Stroke 2004;35:1068–1072.

48 von Reutern GM, von Büdingen HJ: Ultrasound Diagnosis of Cerebrovasclar Disease. Thieme, Stuttgart, 1993.

49 Baumgartner RW, Siebler M: Ultraschalldiagnostik beim Schlaganfall. München, Ecomed-Verlag, 2002.

Dr. David H. Benninger
Department of Neurology, University Hospital
Frauenklinikstrasse 26
CH–8091 Zürich (Switzerland)
Tel. +41 1 255 48 21, Fax +41 1 255 41 41, E-Mail david.benninger@usz.ch

Baumgartner RW, Bogousslavsky J, Caso V, Paciaroni M (eds): Handbook on Cerebral Artery Dissection. Front Neurol Neurosci. Basel, Karger, 2005, vol 20, pp 102–118

Magnetic Resonance Imaging, Magnetic Resonance and Catheter Angiography for Diagnosis of Cervical Artery Dissection

Maurizio Paciaroni, Valeria Caso, Giancarlo Agnelli

Stroke Unit, University of Perugia, Perugia, Italy

Abstract

Catheter angiography has been considered the standard of reference for the diagnosis of spontaneous cervical artery dissection (CAD), but carries a risk of complications and does not demonstrate the arterial wall. The most common angiographic finding is a relatively smooth or slightly irregular tapered arterial narrowing. Conversely, angiographic appearance of cervical artery occlusion due to CAD is nonspecific, because other causes such as thromboembolism or atherosclerotic disease may present very similar angiographic characteristics. Magnetic resonance imaging (MRI) is an alternative noninvasive approach and the only reliable possibility to diagnose occlusive dissection. MRI demonstrates the hyperintense, crescent-shaped wall hematoma and an eccentric flow void of the patent lumen. Intramural hematoma shows a typical evolution of signal intensity over time with intermediate signal intensity on T1-weighted images and high signal intensity on T2-weighted images in the first 3 days. In the following days, most intramural hematoma show slightly or definitively increased signal intensity on T1- and T2-weighted images. After this, signal intensity of the hematoma increases and remains high for approximately 2 months. Magnetic resonance angiography shows the same findings as catheter angiography, and allows in combination with MRI to determine the extent of CAD.

In the last few decades, a major effort has been developed in the research of noninvasive neuroimaging for detecting vascular disease. Although catheter angiography has been considered the gold standard for diagnosing supra-aortic artery dissections, magnetic resonance imaging (MRI) and angiography (MRA) emerge as alternative noninvasive approaches for the diagnosis and monitoring of vertebral (VAD) and internal carotid artery (ICAD) dissections.

The purpose of this chapter is to provide the reader with a basic understanding of the technical aspects of cerebral angiography, MRI, and MRA and their potential for the diagnosis of cervical artery dissection (CAD).

Catheter Angiography

Technical Considerations

Angiography is performed by puncturing the femoral artery and threading a catheter up the iliac artery and into the aortic arch with subsequent selective catheterization of the carotid or vertebral arteries (VA). After entering the desired vessel, an iodine-containing contrast agent is injected and serial films of the vasculature are obtained to demonstrate arterial, capillary, and venous phases of the cerebral circulation. More recently, digital subtraction angiography has been substituted by cut-film angiography, where a computer cancels the background image and transmits it to a television monitor [1]. The advantages are a better image resolution and lower quantity of iodine contrast injected. The potential risks of angiography include minor and major stroke through vessel occlusion and embolic events, contrast reaction, vessel damage (arterial dissection, pseudoaneurysm, and perforation), renal failure, and groin hematoma [2]. The rate of permanent complications is institution dependent and varies between 0.5–0.7% depending on patient risk factors [3, 4]. Risks increase in patients with severe atherosclerosis, advanced age, pre-existing vascular disease, collagen diseases, dysplasias, and acute subarachnoid hemorrhage, as well as with procedure length, quality of catheter, and the amount of contrast used [4]. Relative contraindications for angiography are iodinate contrast media allergy, hypotension, severe hypertension, coagulopathy, renal insufficiency, and congestive heart failure [2].

Catheter Angiography in the Diagnosis of Cervical Artery Dissection

Today, conventional angiography is still considered the standard of reference for the diagnosis of spontaneous ICAD. The angiographic appearance of extracranial ICAD is variable (table 1). The most common finding is a relatively smooth or slightly irregular tapered mid-cervical narrowing [5]. Occlusive dissection is less specific because other causes of occlusion, such as thromboembolism or atherosclerotic disease, present very similar angiographic characteristics (fig. 1). Dissections that occlude the cervical internal carotid artery (ICA) may show a 'rattail' shape (fig. 2). Angiographic demonstration of

Table 1. Angiographic features for diagnosis of CAD

Smooth or slightly irregular tapered narrowing
Occlusion
Rattail-shaped tapered occlusion
Flame-like occlusion
Intimal flap
False or double lumen
Saccular or fusiform aneurysmal dilatation (pseudoaneurysm)
Irregular dilatation

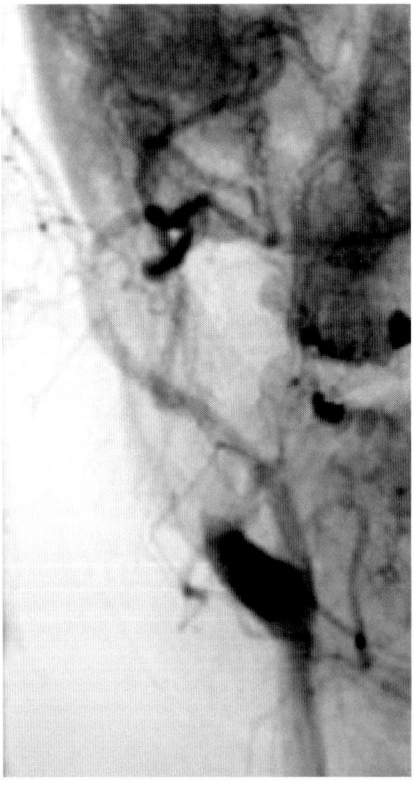

Fig. 1. Catheter angiography shows an occlusion of the internal carotid artery about 2 cm after the origin and a small plaque at the medial wall of the carotid bifurcation. The cause of carotid occlusion was identified by magnetic resonance imaging, which demonstrated a dissection hematoma in the cervical segment of the occluded artery.

an intimal flap or a false lumen is diagnostic but relatively uncommon in spontaneous CAD [6]. A 'flame-like' occlusion, aneurysmal dilatation with or without stenosis or irregularities is also considered to be diagnostic [7] (fig. 3). Angiographic findings depend on the amount of intraluminal thrombus and the extent of the wall hematoma. Pelkonen et al. [8] investigated 76 extracranial

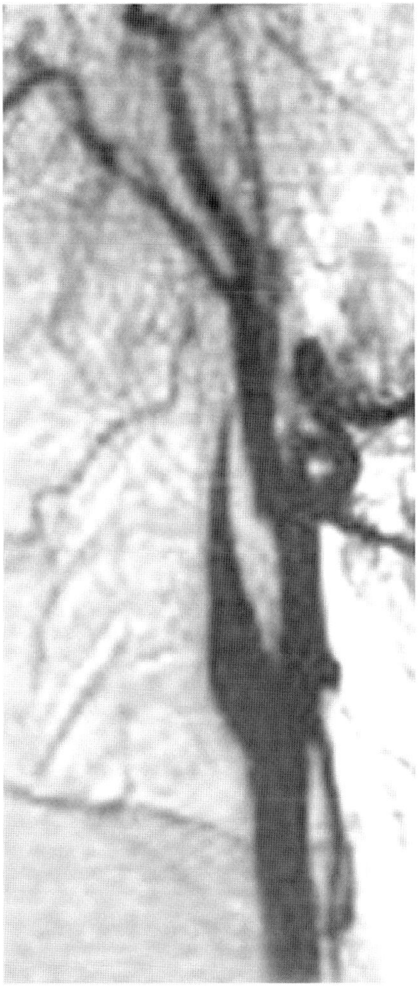

Fig. 2. Catheter angiography shows internal carotid artery dissection with 'rat tail-shaped' occlusion.

ICAD and found 36 (47.4%) irregular stenoses, 22 (28.9%) occlusions, 13 (17.1%) pseudoaneurysms, 4 (5.3%) irregular dilatations, and 1 (1.3%) double lumen. Coexisting ICA kinking or coiling is seen in up to 65% of cases [9]. Pelkonen et al. [8] found in the above-mentioned study 18 kinkings or coilings of the cervical ICA. Dissection affected the redundant vessel segments in 10 cases, while in 4 cases it extended proximally or distally. The dissection was proximal to the kinked or coiled part in 7 cases and distal in one. These data suggest that there is no correlation between the location of the redundancy and the dissected ICA segment.

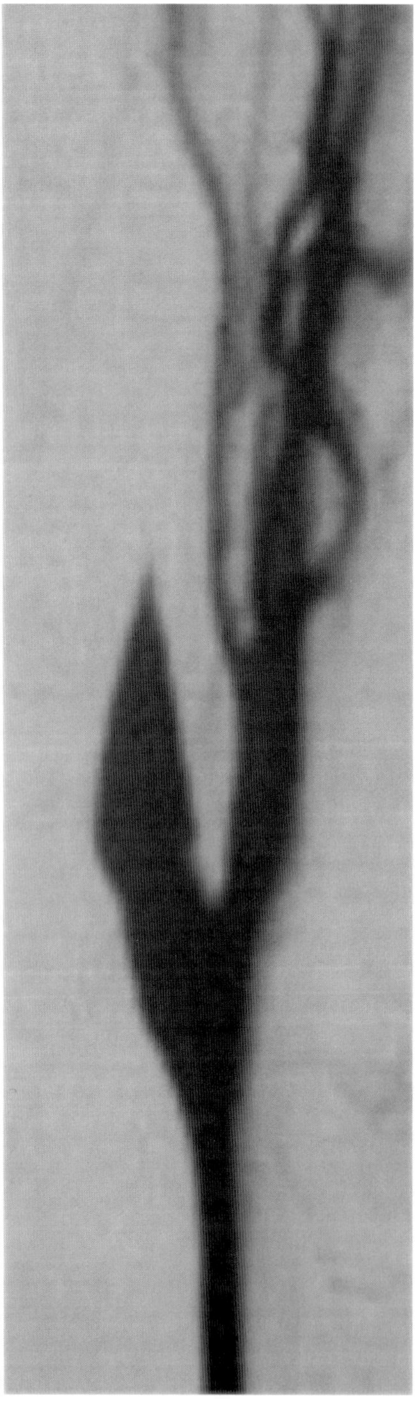

Fig. 3. Catheter angiography shows internal carotid artery dissection with 'flame-like' occlusion. (Courtesy Prof. Ralf W. Baumgartner).

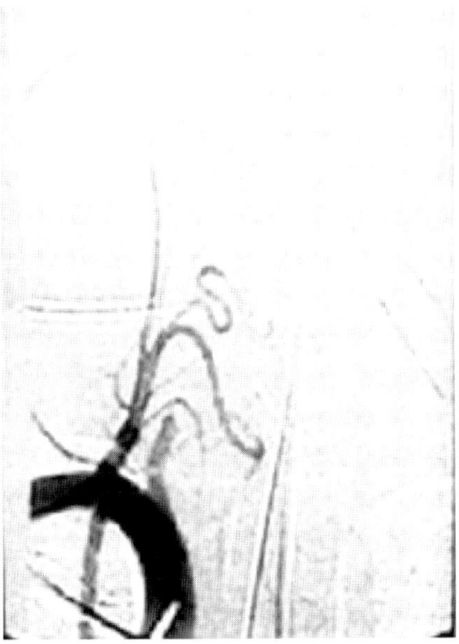

Fig. 4. Catheter angiography shows vertebral artery dissection with tapering occlusion.

ICAD may be caused by a sudden stretching of the ICA over the transverse processes of the upper cervical vertebrae because of hyperextension and flexion or rotation of the neck [10]. Extracranial ICAD affects the cervical part of the artery distal to the carotid bulb [7, 11]. In rare cases the dissection involves the intracranial petrosal segment of the ICA. In this case, MRA is superior in the diagnosis of ICAD (see Magnetic Resonance Imaging and Angiography, p. 108) because a vessel narrowing in this segment is not specific and angiography does not show the arterial wall.

Angiography is still considered the 'gold standard' also for the diagnosis of VAD but is not always definitive in the diagnosis of the disease. Angiography usually reveals indirect, nonspecific signs of VAD, including an elongated or tapered stenosis or pseudoaneurysms; pathognomonic signs such as double lumen or intimal flap are rarely observed as in ICAD. Tapering or abrupt occlusion is a less specific angiographic feature (fig. 4). The angiographic features in patients with spontaneous VAD, in decreasing order of frequency are: luminal stenosis (often irregular and tapered), pseudoaneurysm, occlusion, and intimal flap [12, 13].

VAD may be caused by stretching and compression of the artery over the lateral masses of the first (C1) and second (C2) cervical vertebrae because of hyperextension and flexion or rotation of the neck [14]. This could explain VA involvement at C1–C2 but not at C6–T1 level [8]. Other reports are not consistent regarding the location of VAD; the C1–C6 levels was most frequently affected in one study [15], the C1–C2 level in other studies [8, 12], the level of

C2 and T1 vertebrae in another investigation [16], while a further study failed to establish any preferred site [13].

Angiography is also the better neuroradiological method to evidence filiform stenosis with very slow blood flow, fibromuscular dysplasia, and other irregularities of the vessel wall frequently found in patients with CAD [17].

Magnetic Resonance Imaging and Angiography

Technical Considerations

Some nuclei in the human body become excited when positioned in a strong magnetic field; they absorb the radiofrequency energy of the magnetic field and then release it until they relax completely. The energy is released from the excited tissue over a short period of time according to two relaxation constants known as T1 and T2, and the emitted energy signals are converted into images. The contrasts in the images result from different intensities of the emitted signals, which in turn form different concentrations of the nuclei in different tissues in the body. Hydrogen is the most commonly used nucleus for MRI because of its abundance in biological tissues and the physical properties of the field strengths of the magnets available for clinical use [1]. Other organic particles have been tested but have demonstrated less spatial resolution than hydrogen. The two time constants T1 and T2 are important. T1 is the time constant with which nuclei return to alignment within the static field; T2 is the time constant with which nuclei, all perturbed at the same time by the radiofrequency pulse, lose alignment with each other. T1- and T2-weighted images emphasize different tissue parameters in different ways [18]. In T1-weighted images, tissues with short relaxation time appear bright (methemoglobin, melanin, and fat), whereas tissues with long T1 relaxation times (e.g. cerebrospinal fluid, cyst, edema) appear dark. In T2-weighted images, tissues with long T2 relaxation times (e.g. fluids) appear bright. In general, T1-weighted images provide excellent anatomical details, whereas T2-weighted images provide information about pathological conditions. The fat suppression technique suppresses the normal bright signal of fat on T1-weighted images to improve the visualization of lesions located in fatty areas, such as the neck, orbit, skull base, and spinal canal.

The discovery of the nuclear magnetic resonance phenomenon in bulk matter by Purcell et al. [19] and Bloch et al. [20] in 1946 was rapidly followed by the first observations of the sensitivity of the magnetic resonance experiments regarding flow and motion. The measurement of flow in vivo using phase effects was first reported by Grover and Singer [21] who employed multiple echo sequences with Fourier analysis to study the arterial flow. The first MRA image is attributed to Wedeen et al. [22] in 1985.

MRA is a very sensitive method for detecting and characterizing blood flow based on the physical differences between moving and stationary protons.

Depending on the imaging technique used, blood may appear bright or dark. On traditional MRI, blood vessels usually appear dark. To create bright blood, gradient-echo pulse sequences are used [23]. Bright-blood techniques can be subcategorized into two methods that do not include a contrast agent but generate contrast between flowing blood in a vessel and surrounding stationary tissue [24]. The first and most commonly used method is time-of-flight (TOF) MRA [25], whereas phase contrast (PC) MRA is used less often [26]. TOF techniques generate a positive flow contrast by inflow effects, whereas the background (stationary tissue) is saturated by the rapid repetition of radiofrequency pulses. Use of a segmented gradient-echo sequence with cardiac triggering is helpful for eliminating arterial pulse artifacts [27]. The basis for PC MRA is that the blood flow along a magnetic field gradient causes a shift in the phase of the magnetic resonance signals. PC MRA acquired pairs of images that have different sensitivities to flow. These are then subtracted to cancel background signal, leaving only signals from flowing blood. PC MRA also allows flow (velocity) quantification [28], because the phase shift is proportional to the velocity [23].

For TOF and PC MRA, there are two approaches for data acquisition and image reconstruction: two-dimensional (2D) and three-dimensional (3D) Fourier transformation techniques. 3D MRA produces thinner slices (approximately 0.7–0.8 mm) than 2D MRA (approximately 1.5 mm), which improves spatial resolution and offers more possibilities to study small tortuous vessels, such as the intracerebral arterial circulation [29]. The use of 2D MRA means that the flow/stationary tissue contrast in each slice is always maximal, even with a rather slow flow. The 2D method is therefore appropriate for looking at slow flow such as venous circulation [30], and for acquiring data over a long segment of vessel without saturation effects [31, 32]. This method is also effective for differentiating between slow flow and occlusion. TOF MRA has the disadvantage that the magnetic resonance signal is cancelled when there are disordered fluid flow patterns, such as acceleration or turbulence. This phenomenon is often responsible for the signal loss in an artery at a site of stenosis, marked curvature, or bifurcation. When MRA of supra-aortic vessels is interpreted, special care should be taken to avoid overestimation of stenosis severity in an area of turbulent flow [33, 34]. The tendency of overestimation is reduced in 3D acquisitions, although many neuroradiologists have shown an excellent ability to properly grade severe lesions in 2D TOF [23].

Both 2D and 3D MRA have the disadvantage that stationary material with high signal intensity, such as subacute thrombus, can mimic blood flow. PC MRA is useful in this situation, because the high signal from stationary tissue is eliminated [24]. Compared to the 2D techniques, 3D PC MRA provides a higher spatial resolution and more information on flow direction along each of the three flow-encoding axes (superior-inferior, right-left, and anterior-posterior), but data acquisition time is longer [24]. With sequential 2D or 3D acquisitions, other disadvantages could be possible. Slight patient movement can generate discontinuities in the vessel contour that can mimic a focal stenosis due to fibromuscular dysplasia.

Important advantages have been made recently in MRA by the use of contrast material injection (gadolinium) allowing the acquisition of faster 3D-spoiled gradient-echo pulse sequences (3D contrast-enhanced MRA). The marked shortening of blood related to the contrast material on T1-weighted images allows high signal intensity in vascular structures requiring large imaging volumes. Moreover, flow-related artifacts and in-plane saturation are minimized. The advantage of this technique is that cerebral artery imaging is obtained over a short scanning time of 5–10 min. Data are acquired as the bolus of the gadolinium contrast agent passes through the vessels of interest due to the increased intravascular signal. Vessel signal is determined primarily by gadolinium concentration, analogous to conventional angiography, where vessel detection depends on the concentration of injected contrast. Compared with 2D and 3D TOF MRA, 3D contrast-enhanced MRA delineates carotid stenosis better [35], with high sensitivity (93–100%) and specificity (88–96%), using conventional catheter angiography as the gold standard [36–40].

MRI and MRA in the Diagnosis of CAD

Stenosis or occlusion of an extracranial cerebral artery is not an uncommon finding, and the diagnosis of CAD sometimes cannot be based only on the angiographic appearances described above. In this regard, MRI is especially complementary [41]. By demonstrating a hyperintense, crescent-shaped intramural hematoma and an eccentric flow void of the patent lumen, it confirms the diagnosis of CAD. Intramural hematoma most likely results from intramural hemorrhage through an intimal tear, whereas bleeding of the vasa vasorum seems to be an unlikely mechanism [42]. Until now the question of which sequence is the best to detect the intramural hematoma has not yet been answered. The hematoma shows a typical evolution of signal intensity on repeated MRI, as in intracerebral hemorrhage [43], with intermediate signal intensity on T1-weighted images and high signal intensity on T2-weighted images in the first 3 days (table 2, fig. 5). In the early stages of intramural hemorrhage a hyperintensity on T1-weighted MRI cannot be expected because methemoglobin has not been formed yet. In the following days, most intramural hematoma give slightly or definitively increased signals on T1- and T2-weighted images (fig. 6). After this, the signal intensity of the hematoma

Table 2. Magnetic resonance imaging* features for diagnosis of CAD

Intramural hematoma
First 3 days:
Intermediate signal on T1-weighted images
High signal on T2-weighted images
After 3 days:
Slightly or definitively increased signal on T1- and T2-weighted images
After this the signal intensity of the hematoma increases and remains high for approximately 2 months
In dissection older than 6–12 months, it may be possible to detect an intramural hematoma, which at that stage is isointense with surrounding soft tissue
Eccentric flow void of the patent lumen

*Subacute, hyperintense thrombus is better seen if fat suppression is implemented on T1-weighted acquisitions to eliminate the high signal intensity from perivascular fat tissue.

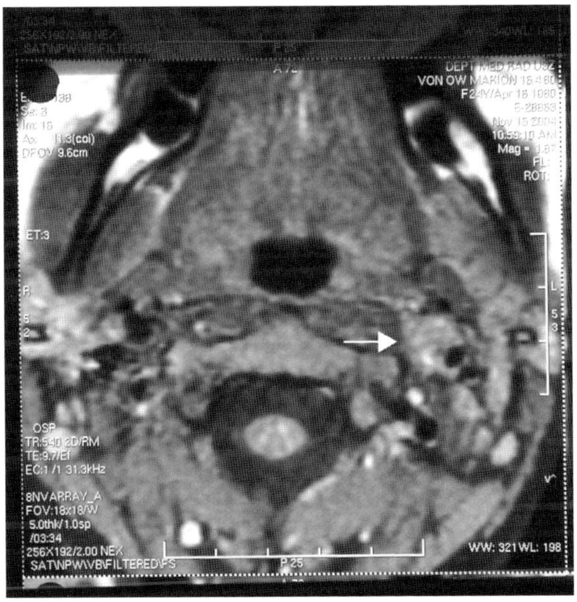

Fig. 5. T1-weighted cervical magnetic resonance imaging with fat-suppression technique of left internal carotid artery dissection shows the intramural hematoma with intermediate signal intensity (white arrow) 2 days after symptom onset (early stage). (Courtesy Prof. Ralf W. Baumgartner).

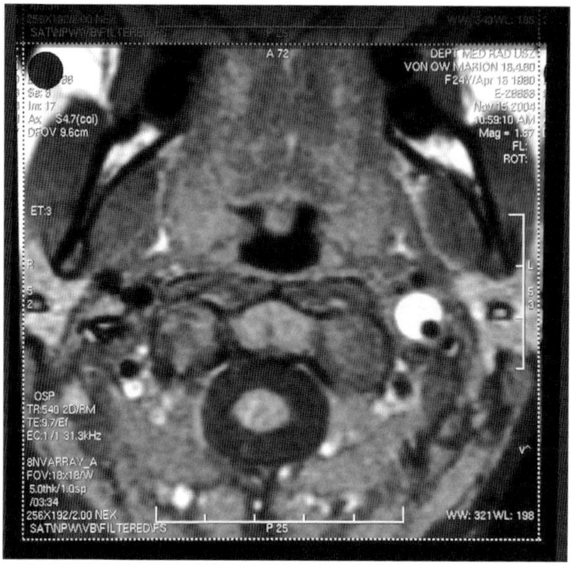

Fig. 6. T1-weighted cervical magnetic resonance imaging with fat-suppression technique of left internal carotid artery dissection shows the intramural hematoma with increased signal intensity six days after symptom onset. (Courtesy Prof. Ralf W. Baumgartner).

increases and remains high for approximately 2 months [44, 45]. If fat suppression is implemented on T1-weighted acquisitions, subacute and hyperintense thrombus are more clearly visualized. In this situation, it is more difficult to detect an intramural hematoma. However, these signal changes are not specific for dissection; fresh thrombus due to atheromatous occlusion may exhibit similar signal evolution and intensity [46]. Nevertheless, crescentic thickening with central signal void proximal to complete occlusion suggests dissection rather than atheromatous occlusion [47, 48]. The shape of a mural hematoma varies according to the relation between the axis of the affected vessel and the imaging plane [49]. Several reports have described crescentic [43, 50], crescent-shaped or oval [51], or circumferential mural hematoma [50]. In dissections older than 2–3 months, the hematoma has been completely dismantled by the surrounding tissue.

To overcome certain limitations of MRI and to increase the sensitivity of noninvasive MR measures, a complimentary MRA is recommended. In fact, when the evaluation includes a 2D- or 3D- TOF combined study or 3D contrast-enhanced MRA, the detection of stenosis, pseudoaneurysm, or occlusion is improved [52, 53] (fig. 7). Additionally, the presence of a thrombosed false lumen is more convincingly demonstrated when spin-echo images are supplemented

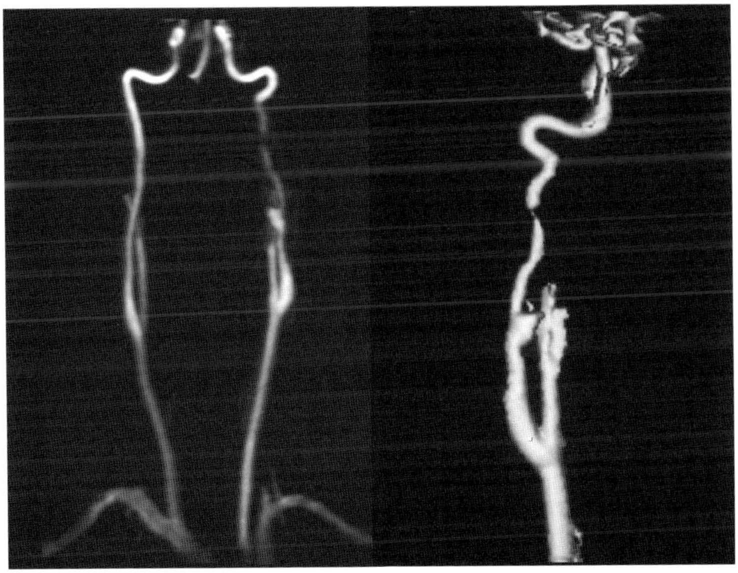

Fig. 7. Magnetic resonance angiography shows internal carotid artery dissection with tapered stenosis and pseudoaneurysm. (Courtesy Prof. Ralf W. Baumgartner).

with PC- or TOF images showing absence of flow in the false lumen [24]. Regarding ICAD involving only a short segment at the cranio-cervical junction can remain undetected if the imaging slabs do not overlap. MRA is superior in revealing the etiology of a petrosal stenosis because of visualization of the arterial wall property [54], while catheter angiography may fail to reveal the etiology of a petrosal stenosis, because vessel narrowing is nonspecific.

3D TOF- or PC MRA combined with MRI allows the diagnosis of dissection and shows its whole extent [55, 56]. Two major advantages of PC MRA in comparison to TOF MRA are the capability to determine the flow direction and to measure the flow velocity [44]. Whereas experience with PC MRA in CAD is limited, the 3D TOF MRA and MRI criteria for diagnosis of CAD are well described and include luminal narrowing or occlusion and an increase of the external artery diameter [47]. An increase in external diameter seems to be the most sensitive sign of ICAD on MRI [5, 47, 55]. However, diagnosis of subacute CAD causing stenosis with TOF-MRA has a potential pitfall [57, 58], as intramural thrombus may not be detected because a high clot signal simulates the flowing blood. This phenomenon is important in stenotic, short dissections, especially in the petrosal segment of the ICA, where no widening of the vessel can be detected. With TOF-MRA, a short dissection, therefore, can easily be missed [54]. Levy et al. [47] describe intramural thrombus in 18/19 ICAD

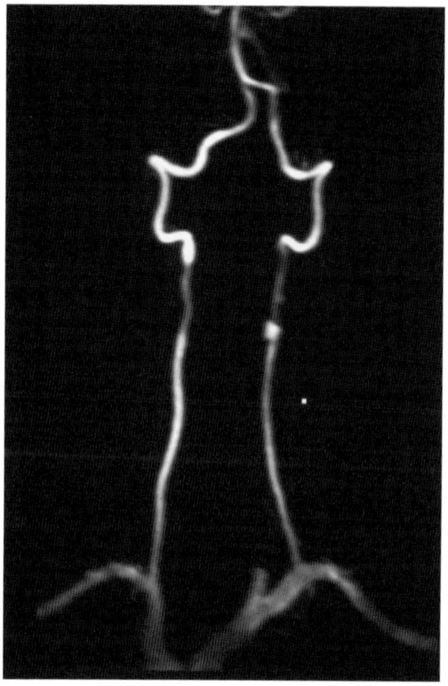

Fig. 8. Magnetic resonance angiography shows bilateral vertebral artery dissection with stenosis and left pseudoaneurysm. (Courtesy Prof. Ralf W. Baumgartner).

(95%) on TOF-MRA. This is due to the signal from the combining of methemoglobin in the intramural clot and the high-flow lumen that both suggest the vessel to be abnormally wide [54].

A high sensitivity (MRA 95%; MRI 84%) and specificity (MRA and MRI 99%) can be obtained in ICAD with 3D TOF MRA and MRI, whereas in VAD a low to moderate sensitivity (MRA 20%; MRI 60%) is accompanied by a high specificity (MRA 100%; MRI 98%) [47]. The greater difficulty in obtaining a correct diagnosis of VAD with MRI and MRA is due to the reduced thickness of the arterial wall, the physiological asymmetries of the small diameter of VAs and high signal intensities of surrounding veins and fat at the cranio-cervical junction [47, 48, 59]. A reduction in arterial lumen alone is a sign with poor specificity as it may be due to hypoplasia, vasospasm, dysplasia without dissection, mere flow reduction, or turbulence [47] (fig. 8). Another nonspecific finding associated with VAD is poor or absent visualization of the VA. Therefore, an altered flow velocity on PC MRA may alone be interpreted as being caused by dissection in conjunction with the detection of a mural hematoma. The normalization or improvement of flow with PC MRA on subsequent investigations favors the diagnosis of dissection [44].

Mascalchi et al. [60] showed that the detection of the VA hematoma on MRI depends on the segment involved. This characteristic reflects the different magnetic resonance signal features of the tissues surrounding the vessel. Dissection at V2 is particularly difficult to identify. In this segment the arterial lumen is often asymmetrical in normal subjects and the artery is surrounded by a small amount of fat giving high signal on T1-weighted images, like a subacute hematoma. Moreover, inflow enhancement phenomena in the venous sinus of the foramen transversarium may mimic a dissection hematoma [47, 61]. Furthermore, Mascalchi et al. [60] noted that intermediate signal from residual slow flow proximal or distal to the dissection can significantly hinder identification of the hematoma especially in the acute phase, when the intramural clot is of intermediate signal intensity on T1-weighted images. Another problem is the common exclusion of V1 from the imaged volume. The authors concluded that MRI is more informative than MRA for diagnosis of spontaneous VAD in the acute phase, with the possible exception of dissection at V2. Regarding the intracranial segment of VA, catheter angiography may be necessary for the correct diagnosis, when finding intramural hematoma on MRI is not satisfactory because angiography is more sensible. The reliability of the typical findings such as double lumen on MRA has not been determined [62].

Conclusions

Intra-arterial conventional angiography has been the standard method for showing the presence and extent of CAD, but carries a risk of complications and does not demonstrate the arterial wall. MRI in association with MRA provides a noninvasive method for investigating CAD, as it allows direct demonstration of an intramural hematoma and enables precise determination of dissection extent. In patients in which the initial MRI and MRA have failed to detect dissection and if clinical history or symptomatology are highly indicative, we suggest implementing these examinations with angiography for primary diagnosis.

References

1 Sklar EML, Ruiz A, Quencer RM, Falcone SF: Neuroimaging. Structural neuroimaging; in Bradley WG, Daroff RB, Fenichel GM, Jankovic J (eds): Neurology in Clinical Practice. Philadelphia, Elsevier, 2004, pp 521–598.

2 Sandhu JS, Wakhloo AK: Neuroimaging. Neuroangiographic anatomy and common cerebrovascular diseases; in Bradley WG, Daroff RB, Fenichel GM, Jankovic J (eds): Neurology in Clinical Practice. Philadelphia, Elsevier, 2004, pp 625–643.

3 Paciaroni M, Caso V, Cardaioli G, Corea F, Milia P, Venti M, Hamam M, Pelliccioli GP, Parnetti L, Gallai V: Is ultrasound examination sufficient in the evaluation of patients with internal carotid artery severe stenosis or occlusion? Cerebrovasc Dis 2003;15:173–176.

4 Willinsky RA, Taylor SM, Terbrugge K, Farb RI, Tomlinson G, Montanera W: Neurologic complications of cerebral angiography: Prospective analysis of 2,899 procedures and review of the literature. Radiology 2003;227:522–528.
5 Provenzale JW: Dissection of the internal carotid and vertebral arteries: Imaging features. AJR Am J Roentgenol 1995;165:1099–1104.
6 Osborn AG: Non atheromatous vasculopathy; in Osborn AG (ed): Diagnostic Cerebral Angiography. Philadelphia, Lippincott Williams and Wilkins, 1999, pp, 342–358.
7 Ast G, Woimant F, Georges B, Laurian C, Haguenau M: Spontaneous dissection of the internal carotid artery in 68 patients. Eur J Med 1993;2:466–472.
8 Pelkonen O, Tikkakoski T, Leinonen S, Pyhtinen J, Lepojarvi M, Sotaniemi K: Extracranial internal carotid and vertebral artery dissections: Angiographic spectrum, course and prognosis. Neuroradiology 2003;45:71–77.
9 Barbour PJ, Castaldo JE, Rae-Grant AD, Gee W, Reed JF 3rd, Jenny D, Longennecker J: Internal carotid artery redundancy is significantly associated with dissection. Stroke 1994;25: 1201–1206.
10 Stringer WL, Kelly DL Jr: Traumatic dissection of the extracranial internal carotid artery. Neurosurgery 1980;6:123–130.
11 Mokri B, Sundt TM Jr, Houser W, Piepgras DG: Spontaneous dissection of the cervical internal carotid artery. Ann Neurol 1986;19:126–138.
12 Mokri B, Houser OW, Sandok BA, Piepgras DG: Spontaneous dissections of the vertebral arteries. Neurology 1988;38:880–885.
13 Provenzale JM, Morgenlander JC, Gress D: Spontaneous vertebral dissection: Clinical, conventional angiographic, CT and MR findings. J Comput Assist Tomgr 1996;20:185–193.
14 Sheth TN, Winslow JL, Mikulis DJ: Rotational changes in the morphology of the vertebral artery at a common site of artery dissection. Can Assoc Radiol J 2001;52:236–241.
15 Chiras J, Marciano S, Molina JV, Touboul J, Poirier B, Bories J: Spontaneous dissecting aneurysm of the extracranial vertebral artery (20 cases). Neuroradiology 1985;27:327–333.
16 Bartels E, Flugen KA: Evaluation of extracranial vertebral artery dissection with duplex-color-flow imaging. Stroke 1996;27:290–295.
17 Schulze HE, Ebner A, Besinger UA: Report of dissection of the internal carotid artery in three cases. Neurosurg Rev 1992;15:61–64.
18 Nolte J (ed): The Human Brain. St. Louis, Mosby, 2002, pp 98–118.
19 Purcell EM, Torrey HC, Pound RV: Resonance absorption by nuclear magnetic moments in a solid. Phys Rev 1946;69:37–38.
20 Bloch F, Hansen WW, Packard M: The nuclear induction experiment. Phys Rev 1946;70:474–485.
21 Grover T, Singer JR: NMR spin-echo flow measurement. J Appl Phys 1971;42:38–40.
22 Wedeen VJ, Meuli R, Edelman RR, Geller SC, Frank LR, Brady TS, Rosen BR: Projective imaging of pulsatile flow with magnetic resonance. Science 1985;230:946–949.
23 Yucel EK, Anderson CM, Edelman RR, Grist TM, Baum Ra, Manning WJ, Culebras A, Pearce W: Magnetic resonance angiography: Update on application for extracranial arteries. Circulation 1999;100:2284–2301.
24 Bowen BC, Saigal G, Ruiz A: Neuroimaging. Computed tomographic and magnetic resonance vascular imaging; in Bradley WG, Daroff RB, Fenichel GM, Jankovic J (eds): Neurology in Clinical Practice. Philadelphia, Elsevier, 2004, pp 599–624.
25 Keller P: Time of flight magnetic resonance angiography. Neuroimaging Clin N Am 1992;4: 639–656.
26 Dumoulin CL: Phase contrast MR angiography techniques. Magn Reson Imaging Clin N Am 1995;3:399–411.
27 Atkinson DJ, Edelman RR: Cineangiography of the heart in a single breath-hold with a segmental turbo FLASH sequence. Radiology 1991;178:357–360.
28 Walker MF, Souza SP, Dumoulin CL: Quantitative flow measurement in phase contrast MR angiography. J Comput Assist Tomogr 1988;12:304–313.
29 Masaryk TJ, Modic MT, Ruggieri PM, Ross JS, Laub G, Lenz CW, Tkach JA, Haacke EM, Selmann WR, Harik SI: Three dimensional (volume) gradient-echo imaging of the carotid bifurcation: Preliminary clinical experience. Radiology 1989;171:801–806.

30 Mattle HP, Wentz KU, Edelman RR, Wallner B, Finn JP, Barnes P, Atkinson DJ, Kleefield J, Hoogewoud HM: Cerebral venography with magnetic resonance. Radiology 1991;178:453–458.

31 Litt AW, Eidelman EM, Pinto RS, Riles TS, McLachlan SJ, Schwartzenberg S, Weinreb JC, Kricheff II: Diagnosis of carotid artery stenosis: Comparison of 2D FT time of flight MR angiography with contrast angiography in 50 patients. Am J Neuroradiol 1991;12:149–154.

32 Graves MJ: Magnetic resonance angiography. Br J Radiol 1997;70:6–28.

33 Urchuk SN, Plewes DB: Mechanisms of flow-induced signal loss in MR angiography. J Magn Reson Imaging 1992;2:453–462.

34 Elgersma OE, Wust AF, Buijs PC, van Der Graaf Y, Eikelboom BC, Mali WP: Multidirectional depiction of internal carotid arterial stenosis: Three dimensional time-of-flight MR angiography versus rotational and conventional digital subtraction angiography. Radiology 2000;216: 511–516.

35 Willig DS, Turski PA, Frayne R, Graves VB, Korosec FR, Swan JS, Mistretta CA, Grist TM: Contrast enhanced 3D MR DSA of the carotid artery bifurcation: Preliminary study of comparison with unenhanced 2D and 3D time-of-flight MR angiography. Radiology 1998;208:447–451.

36 Remonda L, Senn P, Barth A, Arnold M, Lovblad KO, Schroth U: Contrast-enhanced 3D MR angiography of the carotid arteries: Comparison with conventional digital subtraction angiography. AJNR Am J Neuroradiol 2002;23:213–219.

37 Johnston D, Goldstein LB: Clinical carotid endarterectomy decision making: Non invasive vascular imaging versus angiography. Neurology 2001;56:1009–1015.

38 Huston J III, Fain SB, Wald JT, Luether PH, Rydberg CH, Covarrubias DJ, Riederer SJ, Bernstein MA, Brown RD, Meyer PB, Bower TC, Schleck CD: Carotid artery: Elliptic centric contrast-enhanced MR angiography compared with conventional angiography. Radiology 2001;218: 138–143.

39 Lenhart M, Framme N, Volk M, Strotzer M, Manke C, Nitz WR, Finkenzeller T, Feuerbach S, Link J: Time-resolved contrast-enhanced magnetic resonance angiography of the carotid arteries. Diagnostic accuracy and inter-observer variability compared with selective catheter angiography. Invest Radiol 2002;37:535–541.

40 Wutke R, Lang W, Fellner C, Janka R, Denzel C, Lell M, Bautz W, Fellner FA: High-resolution contrast-enhanced magnetic resonance angiography with elliptical centric k-space ordering of supra-aortic arteries compared with selective X-ray angiography. Stroke 2002;33:1522–1529.

41 Kasner SE, Hankins LL, Bratina P, Morgensten LB: Magnetic resonance angiography demonstrates vascular healing of carotid and vertebral artery dissections. Stroke 1997;28: 1993–1997.

42 De Bray JM, Baumgartner RW: History of carotid dissection. Arch Neurol 2005; in press.

43 Goldberg HI, Grosshen R, Gomori J, Asbury AK, Bilaniuk LT, Zimmerman RA: Cervical internal carotid artery dissecting hemorrhage: Diagnosis using MRI. Radiology 1986;158:157–161.

44 Jacobs A, Lanfermann H, Neveling M, Szelies B, Schroder R, Heiss WD: MRI and MRA-guided therapy of carotid and vertebral artery dissections. J Neurol Sci 1997;147:27–34.

45 Gelal FM, Kitis O, Calli C, Yunten N, Vidinli BD, Uygur M: Cranio-cervical artery dissection: Diagnosis and follow-up with MR imaging and MR angiography. Med Sci Monit 2004;10: 109–116.

46 Schwaighofer BW, Klein MV, Lyden PD, Hesselink JR: MR imaging of vertebrobasilar vascular disease. J Comput Assist Tomogr 1990;14:895–904.

47 Levy C, Laissy JP, Raveau V, Amarenco P, Servois V, Bousser MG, Tubiana JM: Carotid and vertebral artery dissection: Three dimensional time of flight MR angiography and MR imaging versus conventional angiography. Radiology 1994;190:97–103.

48 Zuber M, Meary E, Meder JF, Mas JL: Magnetic resonance imaging and dynamic CT scan in cervical artery dissection. Stroke 1993;25:576–581.

49 Auer A, Felber S, Schmidauer C, Waldenberger P, Aichner F: Magnetic resonance angiographic and clinical features of extracranial vertebral artery dissection. J Neurol Neurosurg Psychiatry 64; 474–481.

50 Tobias JA: MRI of intracranial vascular disease with emphasis at low and intermediate field strengths (images at 0.35–1.0T); in Pomeranz SJ (ed): Craniocervical Magnetic Resonance Imaging. Philadelphia, WB Saunders, 1989, pp 315–350.

51 Iwama T, Andoh T, Sakai N, Iwata T, Hirata T, Yamada H: Dissecting and fusiform aneurysm of vertebro-basilar systems: MR imaging. Neuroradiology 1990;32:272–279.
52 Kollias SS, Binkert CA, Ruesch S, Valavanis A: Contrast enhanced MR angiography of the supra-aortic vessels in 24 seconds: A feasibility study. Neuroradiology 1999;41:391–400.
53 Lucas C, Leclerc X, Pruvo JP, Leys D: Dissections arterielle vertebrales: suivi par angiographie par resonance magnetique et injection de gadolinium. Rev Neurol 2000;12:1096–1105.
54 Kirsch E, Kaim A, Engelter S, Lyrer P, Stock KW, Bongartz G, Radu Ew: MR angiography in internal carotid artery dissection: Improvement of diagnosis by selective demonstration of the intramural hematoma. Neuroradiology 1998;40:704–709.
55 Bui LN, Brant-Zawadzki M, Verghese P, Gillan G: Magnetic resonance angiography of cervico-cranial dissection. Stroke 1993;24:126–131.
56 Klufas RA, Hsu L, Barnes PD, Patel MR, Schwartz RB: Dissection of the carotid and vertebral arteries: Imaging with MR angiography. Pictorial assay. Am J Radiol 1995;164:673–677.
57 Sue DE, Brant-Zawadzki MN, Chance J: Dissection of cranial arteries in the neck: Correlation of MRI and arteriography. Neuroradiology 1992;34:273–278.
58 Wagle WA, Dumoulin CL, Souza SP, Cline HE: 3D TOF MR angiography of carotid and basilar arteries. AJNR Am J Neuroradiol 1989;10:911–919.
59 Kitanaka C, Tanaki JI, Kuwahara M, Teraoka A: Magnetic resonance imaging study of intracranial vertebrobasilar artery dissection. Stroke 1994;25:571–575.
60 Mascalchi M, Bianchi MC, Mangiafico S, Ferrito G, Puccioni M, Marin E, Mugnai S, Canapicchi R, Quilici N, Inzitari A: MRI and MR angiography of vertebral artery dissection. Neuroradiology 1997;39:329–340.
61 Miaux Y, Cognard C, Martin-Duverneuil N, Weill A, Savin D, Chiras J: Flow-related enhancement in the vertebral plexus mimicking an intramural hematoma. AJNR Am J Neuroradiol 1996;17: 191–192.
62 Hosoya T, Adachi M, Yamaguchi K, Haku T, Kayama T, Kato Y: Clinical and neuroradiological features of intracranial vertebro-basilar artery dissection. Stroke 1999;30:1083–1090.

Dr. Maurizio Paciaroni
Stroke Unit, University of Perugia, Ospedale Silvestrini
Sant'Andrea delle Fratte
IT–06126 Perugia (Italy)
Tel. +39 075 578 4227/4100, Fax +39 075 578 4227/397153, E-Mail mpaciaroni@libero.it

Baumgartner RW, Bogousslavsky J, Caso V, Paciaroni M (eds): Handbook on Cerebral Artery Dissection. Front Neurol Neurosci. Basel, Karger, 2005, vol 20, pp 119–128

Computed Tomography Angiography for the Evaluation of Carotid Artery Dissections

Christian A. Taschner[a], *Xavier Leclerc*[a], *Christian Lucas*[b], *Jean-Pierre Pruvo*[a]

Departments of [a]Neuroradiology and [b]Neurology, Hôpital Roger Salengro, University Hospital Lille, Lille, France

Abstract

Catheter angiography has long been considered the standard of reference for the diagnosis of cervical artery dissection. The accuracy of magnetic resonance (MR) angiography, Doppler ultrasound or computed tomography angiography (CTA) has been evaluated in a variety of comparative clinical studies. With the development and the increasing propagation of modern multidetector CT techniques, the diagnostic potential of CTA has increased considerably. Our purpose is to summarize the technical aspects and the recent advances of CTA, and to discuss its significance for the diagnosis of cervical artery dissection. In addition the typical CTA appearance of cervical artery dissections is described, and exemplified in various clinical examples. MR angiography remains the method of choice for the exclusion of carotid artery dissection. Multidetector CTA has to be regarded as a safe and reliable diagnostic modality in the evaluation of carotid dissections. But despite its improved quality, the use of CTA in patients with suspected arterial dissection is restricted to a small number of specific indications. At present, its application is reserved for those patients presenting with contraindications to MR imaging.

Catheter angiography has long been considered as the standard of reference for the diagnosis of cervical artery dissection. Due to the invasive character of the method, alternative diagnostic modalities, such as magnetic resonance imaging (MRI), Doppler ultrasound or computed tomography (CT) have been evaluated in clinical studies [1–3]. Among these techniques, MRI has become the method of choice. Advantages of MRI include high spatial resolution allowing direct depiction of the arterial wall and visualisation of the mural hematoma in case of arterial dissection [4–6]. In patients presenting with contraindications for MRI, CT angiography (CTA) can be used alternatively. Previous studies demonstrated the diagnostic potential of helical CT with single detector row for the diagnosis and follow-up of cervical artery dissection [7, 8]. With the development and the increasing propagation of modern multidetector CT techniques, the diagnostic potential of CTA has increased considerably. Our purpose is to summarize the technical aspects and the recent advances of CTA and to discuss its significance for the diagnosis of cervical artery dissection.

Technical Aspects of CTA

Since the invention of the first CT scanner by G.N. Hounsfield in the year 1971, the technology has evolved from a time consuming, expensive technology offering a more than limited image quality to an elegant, fast, and precise tool of modern radiology. Two basic innovations were necessary for this evolutionary process. The introduction of helical CT technology in the beginning of the 1990s significantly reduced the scan time and improved the image quality of CT scans. With the development of multidetector CT technology in the late 1990s, the technology experiences a renaissance.

With helical CT, the radiation source performs a constant rotation around the patient lying on the examination table. During image acquisition, the patient table passes the gantry of the scanner at a constant velocity while detectors measure the penetrating radiation. With first-generation CT scanners, these detectors consisted of scintillation crystals attached to photomultiplier tubes. In our days, gas-filled ionization chambers are applied. With technologies allowing for a reduced gantry rotation time of 0.75–0.8 s, helical CT technology became possible. In contrast to previously applied pencil-shaped X-ray beams and stepwise table feed, a fan-shaped X-ray beam was used, allowing to improve the image quality and to decrease the scanning time. This is particularly useful in patients presenting with difficulties to remain still during the examination. However, the limitations of helical single-beam CT technology need to be addressed. Scan coverage and z-axis coverage/rotation (10 mm) is inadequate to entirely cover the cervical arteries from the aortic arch to the skull base. In addition the resulting anisotropic voxels constrain further postprocessing of image data.

Major advances have been made by the introduction of multidetector CT scans. This new technology allows investigation of a large volume with a high x-axis resolution in a very short time. The basic innovation consist of the application of a cone-shaped X-ray beam, with multiple detector rows receiving the attenuated radiation. This novel approach allows for faster scan coverage and larger z-axis coverage/rotation. With its high spatial resolution and thin slices, the method provides data sets with isotropic voxel size improving the quality of multiplanar reformats and 3D-rendered images.

Multidetector CT has dramatically changed the importance and indications established for CT. Short acquisition times with a very high spatial resolution helped to improve the quality of CTA sustainably. An increasing number of applications are investigated in clinical studies. Multidetector CTA has already been accepted as a means for the evaluation of atherosclerotic carotid disease and for the pretherapeutic evaluation of intracranial aneurysms in clinical practice [9, 10]. So far, the diagnostic potential of multidetector CTA in patients with cervical arterial dissections has not been examined systematically [11].

Imaging Protocol

Pitch, section width, increment, tube current, and voltage are parameters characterizing CT protocols. In single detector row, the pitch is defined as table feed per rotation/nominal slice thickness. In multidetector CT, we are talking about a beam pitch, which is defined as table feed per rotation/nominal slice thickness × number of detector rows. In single detector row CT, a pitch of 1.5 has become the internal standard. This corresponds to pitches of 0.75 in 4-row multidetector CT, 0.875–1.35 at 8-row multidetector CT, and 0.9375–1.375 at 16-row multidetector CT [12]. Higher pitches are usually applied in dynamic imaging, such as perfusion CT [13, 14]. It should be remembered that high pitches are associated with a decrease in z-axis resolution. Multidetector CT allows for acquisition of near-isotropic data sets of overlapping, thinly sliced transverse images. A high-resolution protocol is used for imaging carotid arteries. By using an 8-detector row scanner, a high-resolution 3D volume with a nominal section width of 1.25 mm can be acquired within 10 s [15].

Application of Contrast Media

The intravenous injection of contrast medium (CM) needs to be adapted to faster image acquisition. If applied incorrectly, vessel opacification might be weak, out of phase, or the CM bolus might even be missed completely.

There are different techniques for the administration of CM in multidetector CT imaging: these are measurement of a test bolus, bolus tracking, and continuous injection of contrast. The injection of a small test bolus (10–15 ml) is a reliable means of determining the circulation time with a dynamic, nonincremental CT acquisition. For bolus-triggered application of CM, a region of interest is placed into a target vessel. During the application of CM, nonincremental CT scans are acquired. When a predefined threshold of, for example, 100 HU is obtained, the CT acquisition starts. The triggering delay between passing the threshold in the target vessel and the start of the acquisition depends on the CT scanner used and lies in the range of 2–8 s. After the injection of the CM bolus, saline flushing of the vein is advised as CM can stagnate in the arm veins. Saline flushing improves utilization of CM and enhances the quality of CTA. These two techniques are predominantly applied in multidetector CTA with scanning times below 15 s. For acquisition times longer than 15 s, continuous injection of CM has to be considered. In this case, injection times are usually chosen equaling the scan time. The CM flow rates and the iodine concentration of CM need to be adapted to the demands of fast CTA. A standard flow rate of 4 ml/s of CM with a standard iodine concentration of 300 mg/ml might provide insufficient results as image acquisition can get ahead of CM inflow. The demands of fast CTA are met by using higher inflow rates, or more conveniently, by using CM with a higher density (concentration of iodine >370 mg/ml).

Image Analysis

Image analysis should be performed on a 3D workstation by reviewing the 3D volume data in a dynamic fashion. We recommend becoming comfortable with the transverse sections, because they should be the primary review planes interrogated. Yet, multiplanar reconstructions or curved planar reformats along the vessel axes are available with multidetector CTA. The average level should be preset in the range of 150 HU with a window between 400 and 500 HU.

CTA Imaging at the Acute Phase of Carotid Artery Dissection

Carotid artery dissections usually are confined to the cervical part of the internal carotid artery extending to the skull base. Dissecting disease in most cases spares the carotid bifurcation as well as the intracranial parts of the internal carotid artery.

In the acute phase, carotid artery dissection presents, in 50% of cases, tapered long stenosis on conventional angiograms (fig. 1a) [16]. A typical angiographic feature, encountered in 30% of cases, is the alternation of stenosis followed by dilated segments and the formation of pseudoaneurysms along the affected parts of the artery (fig. 2a) [16]. Carotid artery dissections may finally show occlusive lesions in 20% of cases with a fusiform aspect (fig. 3a) [16].

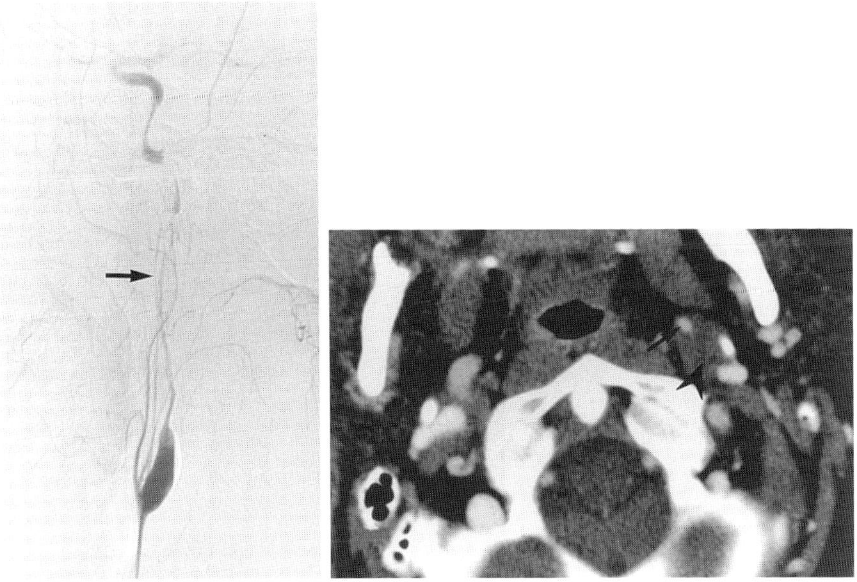

a *b*

Fig. 1. ***a*** Left carotid artery dissection with tapered long stenosis on conventional angiography. ***b*** The external diameter of the carotid artery is enlarged on helical CT, and the arterial lumen appears eccentric (arrow) because of the arterial wall thickening (mural hematoma; arrowhead). The level of the CT slice is indicated on the angiogram (arrow; ***a***).

However, this angiographic appearance is not specific of dissection and may be observed in other circumstances, such as thromboembolic events.

The CTA appearance of carotid artery dissection may differ considerably. Previous studies were able to define various imaging features of carotid artery dissection by using spiral CTA. Carotid artery dissections on CTA may present with occlusion, stenosis, pseudoaneurysm, target picture, mural thickening, or an eccentric arterial lumen. Among these varying modes of presentation, the eccentric arterial lumen seems to be the most reliable indicator of acute dissection (fig. 1b). Mural thickening located at the upper portion of the extracranial internal carotid artery seems to be a highly sensitive and specific sign of carotid artery dissection [7]. Cervical arterial dissection may as well present as an area of arterial wall thickening and a narrowed eccentric lumen surrounded by a thin annular contrast enhancement. This so-called target picture is a very specific, yet less sensitive, sign of arterial dissection (fig. 4). Another fairly reliable criteria for establishing the diagnosis of arterial dissection on CTA is the depiction of an aneurysmally dilated lumen or an alternately dilated and narrowed lumen with or without crescent-shaped mural thickening or an intimal flap (fig. 2b).

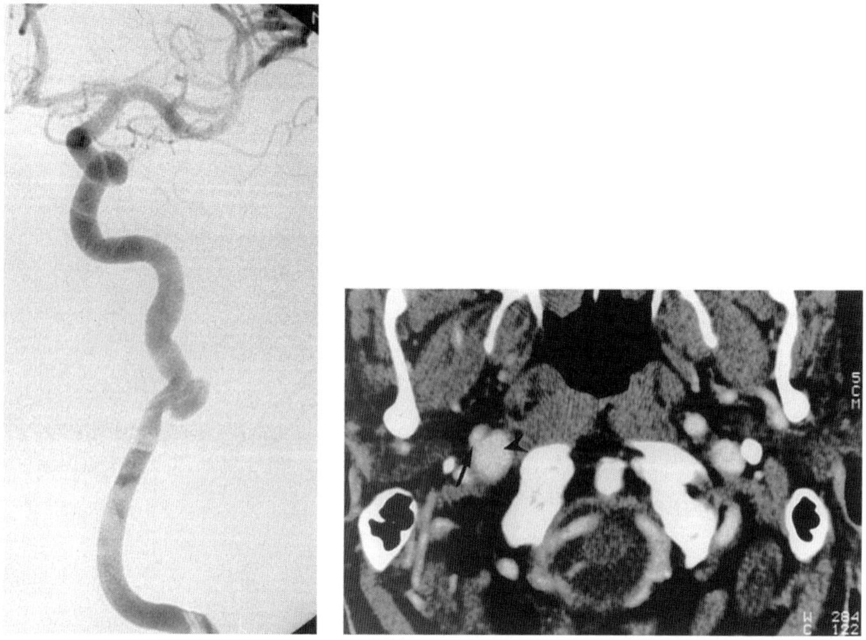

a *b*

Fig. 2. ***a*** Internal carotid artery (ICA) dissection with aneurysm at the upper portion of the right ICA on angiography. ***b*** Helical CT findings showing both narrowed eccentric lumen (arrow) and aneurysm (arrowhead).

The increase of the external diameter of the carotid artery can be established by comparing the diameter at the level of the suspected dissection with either a proximal segment of the internal carotid artery or a corresponding section of the contralateral internal carotid artery (fig. 3b).

CTA in the Follow-Up of Carotid Artery Dissection

On angiographic controls an 'angiographic residuum' has to be expected in about 25% of healed dissections [16]. These residual abnormalities include luminal irregularities related to fibromuscular dysplasia, tortuosities, atheroma, or scar. Previous studies using CTA for the follow-up of patients with cervical artery dissection showed that stenotic-type and nearly occlusive dissections tend to heal with only minor residual mural abnormalities. A disappearance of the aneurysms previously present can be expected in 50–70% of cases [16,17].

CTA is useful for depicting arterial luminal patency after carotid dissection and for showing residual arterial abnormalities – findings that allow physicians a 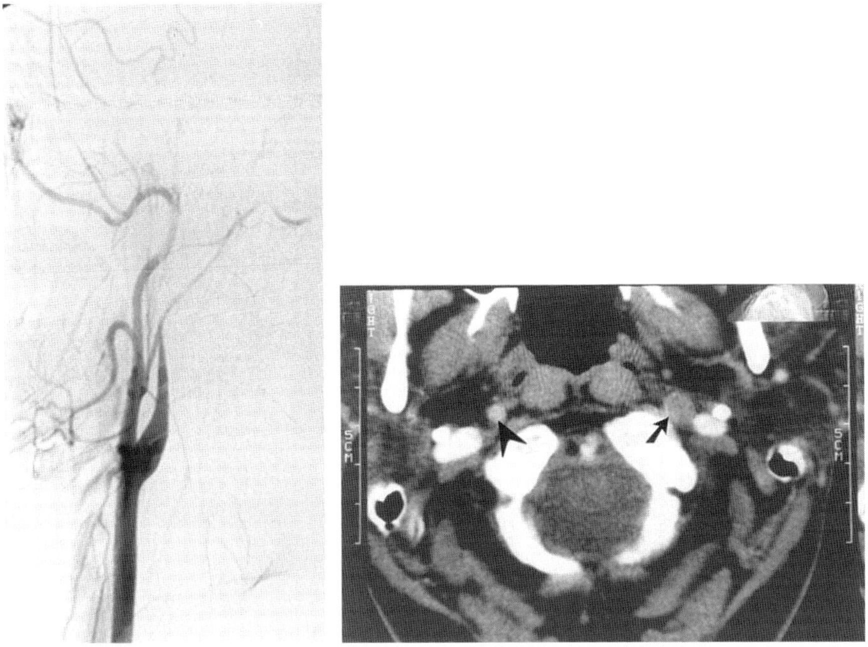 b

Fig. 3. ***a*** Occlusive type dissection of the left internal carotid artery (ICA) on angiography. ***b*** Helical CT demonstrates the increased external diameter (arrow) of the ICA compared with the contralateral side (arrowhead).

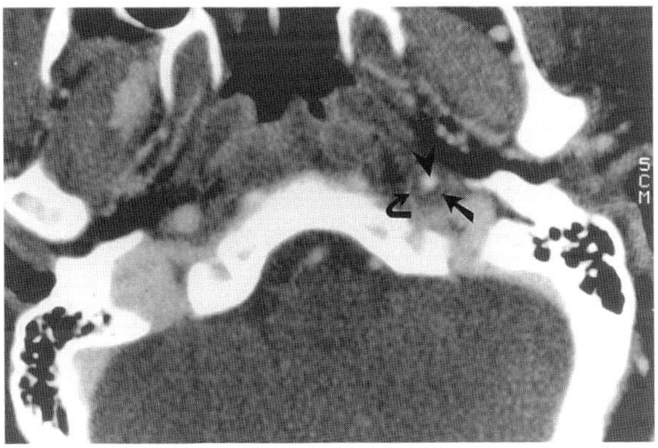

Fig. 4. Typical target CT picture of dissection of the left internal carotid artery associating an arterial wall thickening (straight arrow) with a narrowed eccentric lumen (arrowhead) surrounded by a thin annular contrast enhancement (curved arrow).

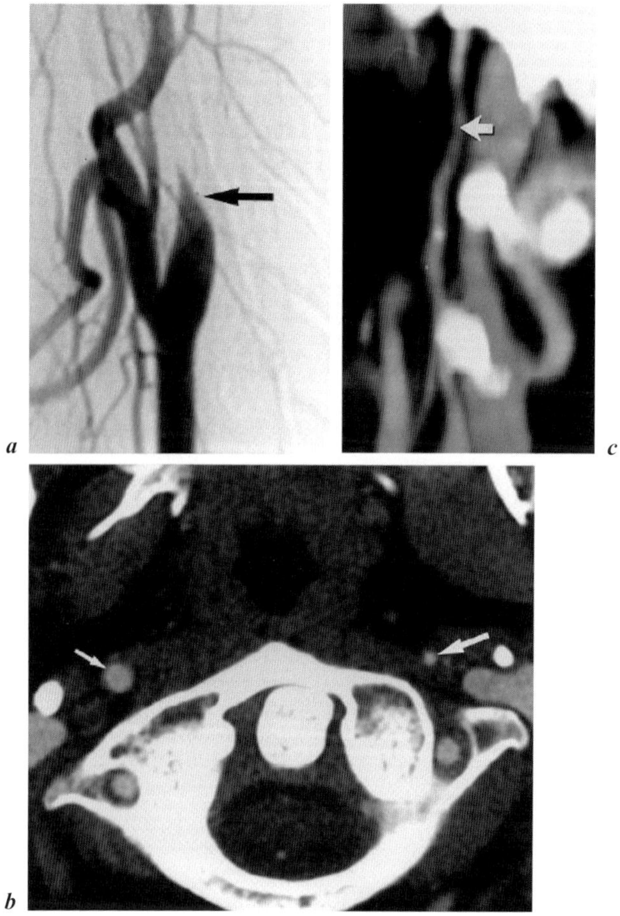

Fig. 5. ***a*** Conventional angiogram 2 days after onset of symptoms reveals complete occlusion of the left ICA with tapered lumen just beyond the bulb (arrow). ***b*** Axial CT scan 3 years later shows a smaller diameter of the left ICA (large arrow) as compared with the contralateral side (small arrow). ***c*** MIP reconstruction shows a severe narrowing throughout the cervical left ICA (arrow).

the flexibility to alter the treatment of ICA dissections as appropriate. Previous studies [8, 18] showed that CTA scans offer good interobserver agreement, and that occlusion, stenosis, and pseudoaneurysms of the cervical ICA are correctly identified (fig. 5). Previous follow-up studies provided results close to those reported for conventional angiography and demonstrated the value of helical CT in monitoring the alterations of extracranial ICA dissections over time.

Discussion

In the past years MR angiography has gradually replaced catheter angiography in the diagnosis of arterial dissection. At present, MR angiography and Doppler ultrasound are considered to be the methods of reference for the diagnostic work-up of patients with suspected arterial dissection. The high sensitivity of CTA for the detection of extracranial dissection has been demonstrated in various studies, and although the quality of CTA has improved dramatically in the past years, it remains a second-line diagnostic tool for the detection of arterial dissections. This is basically due to a couple of limitations inherent to the method. Even with modern multidetector CT scanners, CTA is associated with a radiation dose. In addition, important volumes of iodated CM need to be administered with the risk of contrast reactions. Further drawbacks to CTA are venous contamination, and the limited depiction of smaller vessels embedded into the bone.

Despite its improved quality, the use of CTA in patients with suspected arterial dissection is restricted to a small number of specific indications. With examination times below 20 s, multidetector CTA can be applied in confused and in noncompliant patients. In addition, multidetector CTA has to be regarded as the alternative method of choice in patients that present contraindications to MRI.

Conclusion

MR angiography remains the method of choice for the exclusion of carotid artery dissection. Multidetector CTA has to be regarded as a safe and reliable diagnostic modality in the evaluation of carotid dissections. Its application is reserved for those patients presenting with contraindications to MRI.

References

1 Zuber M, Meary E, Meder JF, Mas JL: Magnetic resonance imaging and dynamic CT scan in cervical artery dissections. Stroke 1994;25:576–581.

2 Provenzale JM: Dissection of the internal carotid and vertebral arteries: Imaging features. AJR Am J Roentgenol 1995;165:1099–1104.

3 Bakke SJ, Smith HJ, Kerty E, Dahl A: Cervicocranial artery dissection. Detection by Doppler ultrasound and MR angiography. Acta Radiol 1996;37:529–534.

4 Levy C, Laissy JP, Raveau V, Amarenco P, Servois V, Bousser MG, Tubiana JM: Carotid and vertebral artery dissections: Three-dimensional time-of-flight MR angiography and MR imaging versus conventional angiography. Radiology 1994;190:97–103.

5 Klufas RA, Hsu L, Barnes PD, Patel MR, Schwartz RB: Dissection of the carotid and vertebral arteries: Imaging with MR angiography. AJR Am J Roentgenol 1995;164:673–677.

6 Kirsch E, Kaim A, Engelter S, Lyrer P, Stock KW, Bongartz G, Radu EW: MR angiography in internal carotid artery dissection: Improvement of diagnosis by selective demonstration of the intramural haematoma. Neuroradiology 1998;40:704–709.
7 Leclerc X, Godefroy O, Salhi A, Lucas C, Leys D, Pruvo JP: Helical CT for the diagnosis of extracranial internal carotid artery dissection. Stroke 1996;27:461–466.
8 Leclerc X, Lucas C, Godefroy O, Tessa H, Martinat P, Leys D, Pruvo JP: Helical CT for the follow-up of cervical internal carotid artery dissections. AJNR Am J Neuroradiol 1998;19:831–837.
9 Wintermark M, Uske A, Chalaron M, Regli L, Maeder P, Meuli R, Schnyder P, Binaghi S: Multislice computerized tomography angiography in the evaluation of intracranial aneurysms: A comparison with intraarterial digital subtraction angiography. J Neurosurg 2003;98:828–836.
10 Jayaraman MV, Mayo-Smith WW, Tung GA, Haas RA, Rogg JM, Mehta NR, Doberstein CE: Detection of intracranial aneurysms: Multi-detector row CT angiography compared with DSA. Radiology 2004;230:510–518.
11 Chen CJ, Tseng YC, Lee TH, Hsu HL, See LC: Multisection CT angiography compared with catheter angiography in diagnosing vertebral artery dissection. AJNR Am J Neuroradiol 2004;25: 769–774.
12 Chawla S: Advances in multidetector computed tomography: Applications in neuroradiology. J Comput Assist Tomogr 2004;28(suppl 1):S12–S16.
13 Roberts HC, Roberts TP, Smith WS, Lee TJ, Fischbein NJ, Dillon WP: Multisection dynamic CT perfusion for acute cerebral ischemia: The ‘toggling-table’ technique. AJNR Am J Neuroradiol 2001;22:1077–1080.
14 Hoeffner EG, Case I, Jain R, Gujar SK, Shah GV, Deveikis JP, Carlos RC, Thompson BG, Harrigan MR, Mukherji SK: Cerebral perfusion CT: Technique and clinical applications. Radiology 2004;231:632–644.
15 Napoli A, Fleischmann D, Chan FP, Catalano C, Hellinger JC, Passariello R, Rubin GD: Computed tomography angiography: State-of-the-art imaging using multidetector-row technology. J Comput Assist Tomogr 2004;28(suppl 1):S32–S45.
16 Houser OW, Mokri B, Sundt TM, Baker HL, Reese DF: Spontaneous cervical cephalic arterial dissection and its residuum: Angiographic spectrum. AJNR Am J Neuroradiol 1984;5:27–34.
17 Quisling RG, Friedman WA, Rhoton AL: High cervical carotid artery dissection: Spontaneous resolution. AJNR Am J Neuroradiol 1980;1:463–468.
18 Marks MP, Napel S, Jordan JE, Enzmann DR: Diagnosis of carotid artery disease: Preliminary experience with maximum intensity projection spiral CT angiography. AJR Am J Roentgenol 1993;160:1267–1271.

Dr. Christian A. Taschner
Department of Neuroradiology
Hôpital Roger Salengro, University Hospital Lille
FR–59037 Lille (France)
Tel. +33 3 20 446468, Fax +33 3 20 446488, E-Mail c.taschner@web.de

Baumgartner RW, Bogousslavsky J, Caso V, Paciaroni M (eds): Handbook on Cerebral Artery Dissection. Front Neurol Neurosci. Basel, Karger, 2005, vol 20, pp 129–139

Prognosis of Cervical Artery Dissection

Emmanuel Touzé, Jean-Yves Gauvrit, Jean-François Meder, Jean-Louis Mas

Service de Neurologie, Hôpital Sainte-Anne, Paris, France

Abstract

The prognosis of cervical artery dissection (CAD) patients mainly depends on the severity of the initial stroke and the risk of subsequent stroke. The overall functional prognosis of patients with stroke due to CAD does not differ from that of young patients with stroke due to other causes. The annual risk of recurrent stroke ranges from 0.3 to 3.4%. Early recurrences are often in the territory of the CAD when arterial lesions had not completely recovered. Conversely, long-term recurrent ischemic events seem to take place in all territories and can be due to various mechanisms. The prognosis of CAD patients also depends on the arterial outcome. Stenotic lesions resolve within a few months, most often without visible sequel on angiogram, in about 70% of patients. Recanalization of occluded vessels is less frequent but in more recent studies, which used imaging to confirm the presence of a mural hematoma, recanalization occurred in up to 90% of cases. Carotid aneurysms persist in about two third of cases while vertebral aneurysms seem to frequently resolve. Complications related to persistent aneurysm seem to be exceptional. The overall risk of CAD recurrence is low, ranging from 0.3 to 1.4% but seems to be higher within the first month and some recurrences are asymptomatic. Patients with connective tissue disease or familial history of CAD have an increased risk of CAD recurrence, but other risk factors remain unknown.

The prognosis of cervical artery dissection (CAD) consists at first of the neurological outcome, which is related to the severity of the initial ischemic insult and to the risk of subsequent stroke. It also consists of the arterial outcome, which corresponds to the evolution of the arterial lesions and the subsequent risk of CAD recurrences. Very early reports, often based on autopsy studies, associated CAD with a high mortality rate [1]. Recent publications have shown that patients who survive the initial episode usually improve or recover [2, 3]. So far, studies devoted to the long-term risk of recurrent events

Table 1. Neurological outcome of stroke after cervical artery dissection

Reference (year of publication)	Patients, n	Death in the acute phase, %	Follow-up, years	Survivors with good/excellent outcome, %
Mokri and Sundt [2] (1986)	36	0	4.9	72
Bogousslavsky et al. [4] (1987)	30	23	3.2	52
Mokri et al. [13] (1988)	25	0	3.8	88
D'Anglejan et al. [3] (1990)	62	1.6	3.4	71
Pozatti et al. [39] (1990)	19	16	8.2	44
Ast et al. [11] (1993)	68	1.5	1.0	42
Leys et al. [6] (1995)	110	ND	3.0	73
Engelter et al. [50] (2000)	33	3	2.3	78
Beletsky et al. [8] (2003)	116	ND	1.0	86

ND = Not described.

have been quite rare [4–8]. Many uncertainties persist with regards to the influence of antithrombotic drugs on the ischemic events risk.

Neurological Prognosis

Functional Prognosis and Persistent Headaches

The clinical manifestations of CAD include transient ischemic attacks (TIA), stroke, and local signs and symptoms, which can occur in combination or in isolation. Most patients with ischemic complications have preceding local manifestations. However, as many patients with isolated local signs are underdiagnosed, the absolute risk of ischemic complications beyond the onset of local manifestations is unknown. In patients with stroke or TIA, the delay between the first symptoms of CAD and ischemic event widely varies from few minutes to one month. However, most strokes occur within the first week [9]. The functional prognosis of patients with stroke mainly depends on the size and the localization of the infarct [10]. The reported rate of death from dissections of the carotid and vertebral arteries is very low in most case series (table 1) [2, 4, 5, 9, 11–13]. However, this rate is probably underestimated because patients admitted in a critical neurological state do not always have arterial examinations allowing the diagnosis of CAD. Actually, CAD constitutes a potential cause of massive or malignant middle cerebral artery infarct in young subjects resulting from acute carotid occlusion. For example, in a series of 63 patients with malignant middle cerebral artery infarct, 19 (30%) had a CAD [14].

Among patients who survived a stroke due to CAD, a fairly good neurological prognosis is noted in about three fourths of adult cases (table 1). Children also seem to have a favorable outcome after a dissection although very few cases have been reported [15]. However, the overall functional prognosis of patients with stroke due to CAD does not seem to significantly differ from that of young patients with stroke due to other causes [16, 17]. It has been suggested that patients with traumatic dissection may have more severe long-term neurological deficits than those with spontaneous dissection, but this finding did not receive any clear explanation [18].

Headache and cervical pain occur in up to 75% of patients with CAD and may be the only clinical manifestation [19]. In addition, migraine, which is a risk factor for CAD, is present in about 50% of patients before CAD [20–22]. After a CAD, a dramatic improvement or worsening of migraine can be observed. Moreover, some patients without past history of migraine have residual headache, which sometimes fulfill criteria for migraine [6]. In the study of Leys et al. [6], about one third of patients with post-CAD headache complained of pain spreading to the ipsilateral cervical area. The mechanisms of such headache and cervical pain remain unknown. Persistent pain is observed in patients without ischemic symptoms, as well as in those with brain infarct, suggesting that pain is more likely linked to the arterial involvement than the brain lesion.

Recurrent Ischemic Events

Table 2 summarizes results of the studies devoted to the prognosis of CAD. The annual risk of recurrent stroke ranges from 0.3 to 3.4% and that of TIA from 0.6 to 1.7% [3–8, 23–25]. Stroke and TIA, which occur after a CAD, can result from recurrent CAD (see below), persistent arterial lesion (occlusion, stenosis, aneurysm) or other common causes of stroke in young subjects. Recurrent events seem to be more frequent during the first weeks of CAD [7, 8]. Those early recurrences are often in the territory of the CAD when arterial lesions had not completely recovered [7]. Conversely, ischemic events occurring during long-term follow-up seem to take place in all territories and can be due to various mechanisms. In the muticenter study conducted in France (459 patients followed up for a mean of 31 months), 4 (2 strokes and 2 TIA) out of the 12 ischemic events occurred within the 6 months of the qualifying event and were due to persistent acute CAD. Beyond 6 months, 8 ischemic events (2 strokes and 6 TIA) were observed. Both strokes were due to a contralateral recurrent dissection. Of the 6 late TIA, 3 occurred in the territory of the initial CAD and 3 TIA in an undetermined territory [7]. One patient had persistent

Table 2. Long-term risk of ischemic events and recurrence in cervical artery dissection

Reference (year of publication)	Country	Patients (survivors), n	Anatomical subtype	Follow-up, years	Annual risk, %		
					ischemic stroke	TIA	recurrent CAD
Bogousslavsky et al. [4] (1987)	Switzerland	24	ICAD	3.2	1.3	0	1.3
D'Anglejan et al. [3] (1990)	France	59	ICAD	3.4	ND	ND	0.9
Pozatti et al. [39] (1990)	Italy	16	ICAD, occlusion	8.2	0	0	0
Schievink et al. [5] (1994)	USA	199	ICAD and VAD	7.4	ND	ND	1.1
Leys et al. [6] (1995)	France	105	ICAD and VAD	3.0	0.6	1.0	1.0
Bassetti et al. [23] (1996)	Switzerland	74	ICAD and VAD	2.8	ND	ND	1.4
Guillon et al. [29] (1999)	France	16	ICAD with aneurysm	3.0	0	0	0
Engelter et al. [50] (2000)	Switzerland	33	ICAD	2.3	2.7	1.4	0
Touzé et al. [21] (2001)	France	35	ICAD and VAD with aneurysm	3.5	0	0	0
Touzé et al. [7] (2003)	France	459	ICAD and VAD	2.6	0.3	0.6	0.3
Beletsky et al. [8] (2003)	Canada	116	ICAD and VAD	1.0	3.4	1.7	0
Kremer et al. [25] (2003)	Switzerland	92	ICAD with severe stenosis or occlusion	6.7	1.1	1.0	0.6

ICAD = Internal carotid artery dissection; ND = not described; VAD = vertebral artery dissection.

carotid stenosis and etiology was undetermined in the 5 remaining TIA [7]. The prospective Canadian study also suggested that recurrent events mostly occur in the first weeks after dissection, but deaths, which may also be due to the initial stroke, were included in recurrent events [8].

Exceptional cases of stroke in patients with chronic carotid aneurysm retrospectively attributed to an ancient and missed CAD have been reported [26, 27]. Stroke was usually attributed to thrombus migration from the aneurysm, sometimes found during surgical procedure [28]. However, in two prospective studies specifically devoted to patients with persistent carotid or carotid and vertebral aneurysm after a CAD, no event was observed [21, 29]. The stroke risk seems also to be low in patients with persistent severe stenosis or occlusion (table 2) [25]. These findings do not support the use of invasive therapies such as surgery [30–32] or endovascular procedures [33–35] in the vast majority of patients with persistent arterial lesions after a CAD [21, 25, 29]. Conservative management with antiplatelet therapy seems a prudent strategy, and invasive options should be only proposed in patients with recurrent events despite well-conducted medical therapies.

Arterial Prognosis

Evolution of Arterial Lesions

Improvement of arterial lesions of dissection over time is the rule and may constitute a strong argument for the diagnosis of CAD [1]. Interestingly, worsening of the arterial lesion during the acute phase of dissection has been reported sometimes, but this unusual evolution most often has no clinical counterpart [36]. The long-term anatomical outcome seems to depend on the initial angiographic form. Stenotic lesions resolve within a few months, most often without visible sequel on angiogram, in about 70% of patients (fig. 1) [2, 3, 6, 13, 25, 37, 38]. Recanalization of occluded vessels seems less frequent. In old series, which only used angiography, recanalization occurred in about 40% of patients [2, 4, 37, 39]. Yet, in more recent studies, which used MRI, duplex sonography or CT scan to confirm the presence of a mural hematoma, recanalization occurred in up to 90% of cases, suggesting that older studies included occlusions which were not due to CAD [40, 41]. Recanalization usually occurs within the first weeks and seems to be exceptional beyond 3 months. Recanalization does not influence neurological outcome [42]. The frequency of aneurysmal forms of CAD ranges from 13 to 49% for ICA [2, 3, 11, 18, 21, 29, 37, 40] and from 10 to 46% for VA [12, 13, 21, 43]. Aneurysm can be associated with stenotic form or can constitute the evolution of an occlusive form (fig. 2). It should be pointed out that some aneurysms may be missed if only an

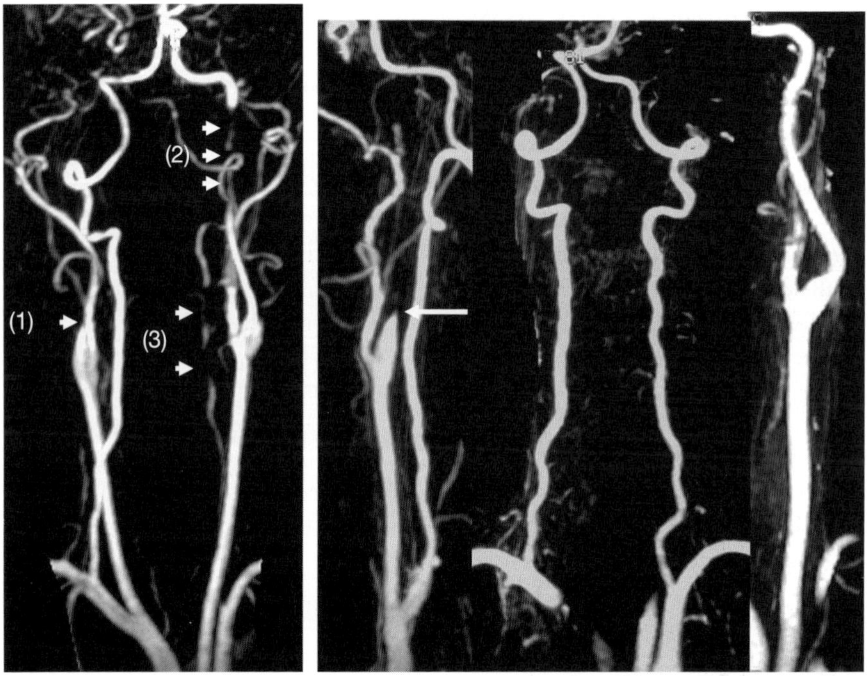

a b

Fig. 1. Multiple cervical artery dissection: ***a*** Initial evaluation: occlusion of right internal carotid artery (1), stenoses of left internal carotid (2) and vertebral arteries (3). ***b*** Follow-up (3 months): persistence of right carotid artery occlusion (arrow), and resolution of left carotid and vertebral artery stenoses.

acute stage angiography is performed, because blood flow distal to the stenosis may be insufficient to fulfill the aneurysm at the acute phase [21]. Two studies specifically devoted to the outcome of aneurysmal forms of CAD have found that aneurysms of the internal carotid artery frequently persist [21, 29]. Guillon et al. [29] found that 95% (out of 20) carotid aneurysms persisted after a 3-year mean follow-up. Touzé et al. [21] found that 64% (out of 33) carotid aneurysms persisted after a 3.5-year mean follow-up. Anatomical outcome of vertebral aneurysms seems better than that of carotid ones since only 17% of the 9 aneurysms persisted in the latter study. In both studies, no increase in aneurysm size was observed at follow-up angiographies, mainly magnetic resonance angiography, and no patients had clinical complications (ischemic events, mass effect or rupture). Aneurysm involving an asymptomatic artery is sometimes found at the acute phase of CAD. Whether this aneurysm represents a previous dissection and has been present for many years or represents a purely aneurysmal form of acute CAD remains uncertain. However, these aneurysms rarely

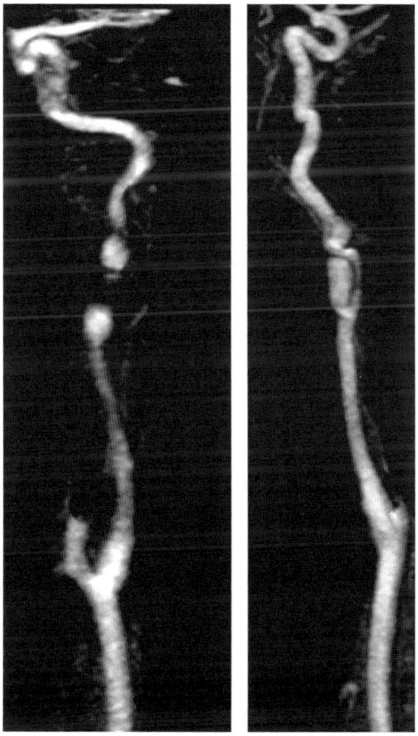

a b

Fig. 2. Carotid artery dissection (aneurysmal form). ***a*** Initial evaluation showing severe stenosis and aneurysms. ***b*** Follow-up evaluation showing an improvement of the stenosis but persistence of aneurysms.

seem to disappear, suggesting that they are most often due to a previous silent dissection [21].

Risk of Recurrent CAD

The overall risk of CAD recurrence is low, ranging from 0.3 to 1.4% (table 2) but seems to be higher within the first month [5]. Indeed, Schievink et al. [5] found a risk of CAD recurrence of 2% in the first month and of 1% beyond. Besides, early CAD recurrences could be underestimated, because asymptomatic recurrences could be more frequent than symptomatic ones (fig. 3) [44] Risk factors for CAD recurrence are not well known. Patients with connective tissue disease or familial history of CAD have an increased risk of CAD recurrence [5, 6, 45–47]. Schievink et al. [46] found an increased risk of CAD recurrence in patients with a familial history of dissection (RR, 6.3; 95% CI, 2.2–18.3%) which corresponded to an absolute risk of 50 vs. 5.8%. In the study of Leys et al. [6], 2 of the 3 patients with CAD recurrence had connective tissue

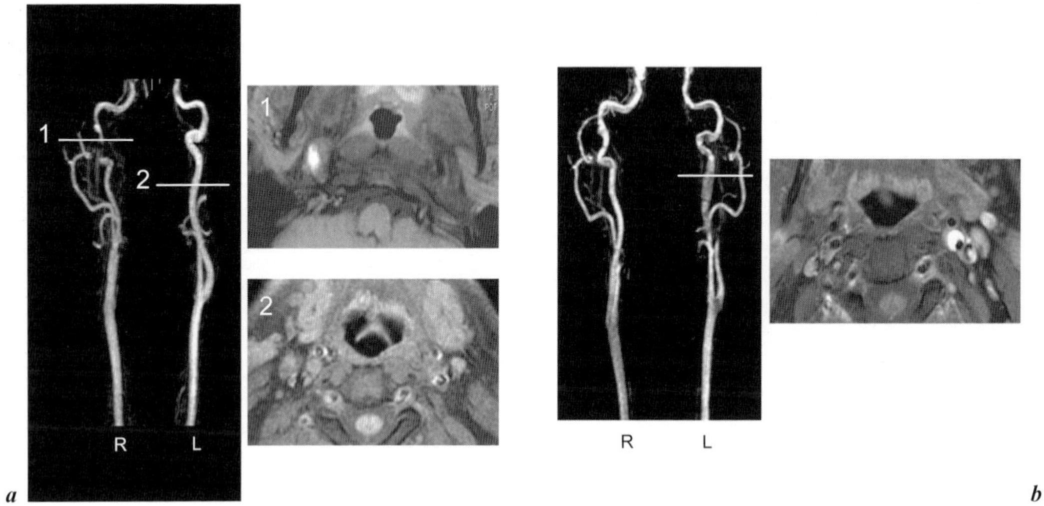

Fig. 3. Asymptomatic early recurrence. ***a*** Initial evaluation: right internal carotid artery stenosis. ***b*** Follow-up evaluation: resolution of right carotid stenosis but occurrence of asymptomatic aneurysmal form of dissection of the left internal carotid artery.

disease. Nevertheless, familial dissections and connective tissue diseases are exceptional in practice. The low prevalence of connective tissue disease observed in the multicenter study conducted in France possibly explains the low risk of CAD recurrences [7]. Thus, the risk of recurrence is probably under 1% per year in patients without severe connective tissue disease.

Role of Antithrombotic Treatments

Although their efficacy has never been established, anticoagulants are widely used in the acute phase of CAD [48]. Heparin is usually administered in the acute phase, and then replaced by oral anticoagulants for a mean period of 3 months. This attitude is justified by the fact that most strokes seem to result from thromboembolic mechanism [49]. One recent prospective observational study performed in 105 patients with CAD found a nonsignificant trend that the rate for recurrent TIA and ischemic stroke or death was higher in patients treated with aspirin (12.4%) than with anticoagulation (8.3%) [8]. A retrospective study did not find any difference in the risk of ischemic events between patients under anticoagulants and those under aspirin [50]. In addition to the risk of intracranial or systemic hemorrhage, anticoagulants carry a theoretical risk of worsening the intramural hematoma [1]. However, this negative effect is not confirmed by everyday practice. The question of whether anticoagulants are better than aspirin in the prevention of early recurrent events can be answered by a therapeutic trial that would require about 2,000 patients [8]. Beyond the acute phase, anticoagulants are frequently relayed by an antiplatelet treatment. The benefit of antithrombotic drugs in the prevention of long-term ischemic events after a CAD has never been assessed. In studies devoted to the prognosis of patients with persistent arterial lesions, most patients received antiplatelet drugs. Many practitioners advise to continue antiplatelet drugs in patients who keep arterial abnormalities (e.g., stenosis, aneurysm) and to stop these drugs in those who have a complete recovery of their dissection. The very low risk of long-term ischemic events, even in patients with persistent arterial lesions, makes it difficult to evaluate the long-term benefit of antithrombotic drugs after a CAD. There is no reason to believe that antithrombotic drugs could reduce the risk of CAD recurrence.

References

1 Hart RG, Easton JD: Dissections of cervical and cerebral arteries. Neurol Clin 1983;1:155–182.
2 Mokri B, Sundt TM Jr, Houser OW, Piepgras DG: Spontaneous dissection of the cervical internal carotid artery. Ann Neurol 1986;19:126–138.
3 D'Anglejan Chatillon J, Ribeiro V, Mas JL, Bousser MG, Laplane D: Dissection de l'artère carotide interne extracrânienne: 62 cases. Presse Med 1990;19:661–667.
4 Bogousslavsky J, Despland PA, Regli F: Spontaneous carotid dissection with acute stroke. Arch Neurol 1987;44:137–140.
5 Schievink WI, Mokri B, O'Fallon WM: Recurrent spontaneous cervical-artery dissection. N Engl J Med 1994;330:393–397.
6 Leys D, Moulin T, Stojkovic T, Begey S, Chavot D: Follow-up of patients with history of cervical artery dissection. Cerebrovasc Dis 1995;5:43–49.
7 Touzé E, Gauvrit JY, Moulin T, Meder JF, Bracard S, Mas JL: Risk of stroke and recurrent dissection after a cervical artery dissection: A multicenter study. Neurology 2003;61:1347–1351.
8 Beletsky V, Nadareishvili Z, Lynch J, Shuaib A, Woolfenden A, Norris JW: Cervical arterial dissection: Time for a therapeutic trial? Stroke 2003;34:2856–2860.
9 Biousse V, D'Anglejan-Chatillon J, Touboul PJ, Amarenco P, Bousser MG: Time course of symptoms in extracranial carotid artery dissections. A series of 80 patients. Stroke 1995;26:235–239.
10 Adams HP, Love BB, Jacoby R: Arterial dissections; in Ginsberg MD, Bogousslavsky J (eds): Cerebrovascular Disease. Oxford, Blackwell Sciences, 1998, pp 1430–1446.
11 Ast G, Woimant F, Georges B, Laurian C, Haguenau M: Spontaneous dissection of the internal carotid artery in 68 patients. Eur J Med 1993;2:466–472.
12 Mas JL, Bousser MG, Hasboun D, Laplane D: Extracranial vertebral artery dissections: A review of 13 cases. Stroke 1987;18:1037–1047.
13 Mokri B, Houser OW, Sandok BA, Piepgras DG: Spontaneous dissections of the vertebral arteries. Neurology 1988;38:880–885.
14 Schwab S, Steiner T, Aschoff A, Schwarz S, Steiner HH, Jansen O, Hacke W: Early hemicraniectomy in patients with complete middle cerebral artery infarction. Stroke 1998;29:1888–1893.
15 Schievink WI, Mokri B, Piepgras DG: Spontaneous dissections of cervicocephalic arteries in childhood and adolescence. Neurology 1994;44:1607–1612.
16 Leys D, Bandu L, Henon H, et al: Clinical outcome in 287 consecutive young adults (15 to 45 years) with ischemic stroke. Neurology 2002;59:26–33.

17 Kappelle LJ, Adams HP Jr, Heffner ML, Torner JC, Gomez F, Biller J: Prognosis of young adults with ischemic stroke. A long-term follow-up study assessing recurrent vascular events and functional outcome in the Iowa Registry of Stroke in Young Adults. Stroke 1994;25:1360–1365.
18 Mokri B: Traumatic and spontaneous extracranial internal carotid artery dissections. J Neurol 1990;237:356–361.
19 Biousse V, Woimant F, Amarenco P, Touboul PJ, Bousser MG: Pain as the only manifestation of internal carotid artery dissection. Cephalalgia 1992;12:314–317.
20 D'Anglejan-Chatillon J, Ribeiro V, Mas JL, Youl BD, Bousser MG: Migraine – A risk factor for dissection of cervical arteries. Headache 1989;29:560–561.
21 Touzé E, Randoux B, Meary E, Arquizan C, Meder JF, Mas JL: Aneurysmal forms of cervical artery dissection: Associated factors and outcome. Stroke 2001;32:418–423.
22 Tzourio C, Benslamia L, Guillon B, Aidi S, Bertrand M, Berthet K, Bousser MG: Migraine and the risk of cervical artery dissection: A case-control study. Neurology 2002;59:435–437.
23 Bassetti C, Carruzzo A, Sturzenegger M, Tuncdogan E: Recurrence of cervical artery dissection. A prospective study of 81 patients. Stroke 1996;27:1804–1807.
24 Baumgartner RW, Arnold M, Baumgartner I, Mosso M, Gonner F, Studer A, Schroth G, Schuknecht B, Sturzenegger M: Carotid dissection with and without ischemic events: Local symptoms and cerebral artery findings. Neurology 2001;57:827–832.
25 Kremer C, Mosso M, Georgiadis D, Stockli E, Benninger D, Arnold M, Baumgartner RW: Carotid dissection with permanent and transient occlusion or severe stenosis: Long-term outcome. Neurology 2003;60:271–275.
26 Mokri B, Piepgras DG, Sundt TM, Pearson BW: Extracranial internal carotid artery aneurysms. Mayo Clin Proc 1982;57:310–321.
27 Peeters A, Goffette P, Dorban S, Sindic JM, Cosnard G: An old dissecting aneurysm of the internal carotid artery presenting as acute stroke. Acta Neurol Belg 2003;103:179–182.
28 Mokri B, Piepgras DG, Houser OW: Traumatic dissections of the extracranial internal carotid artery. J Neurosurg 1988;68:189–197.
29 Guillon B, Brunereau L, Biousse V, Djouhri H, Levy C, Bousser MG: Long-term follow-up of aneurysms developed during extracranial internal carotid artery dissection. Neurology 1999;53:117–122.
30 Candon E, Marty-Ane C, Pieuchot P, Frerebeau P: Cervical-to-petrous internal carotid artery saphenous vein in situ bypass for the treatment of a high cervical dissecting aneurysm: Technical case report. Neurosurgery 1996;39:863–866.
31 Coffin O, Maiza D, Galateau-Salle F, Martel B, Vignon C, Neri E, Derlon JM: Results of surgical management of internal carotid artery aneurysm by the cervical approach. Ann Vasc Surg 1997;11:482–490.
32 Schievink WI, Piepgras DG, McCaffrey TV, Mokri B: Surgical treatment of extracranial internal carotid artery dissecting aneurysms. Neurosurgery 1994;35:809–815.
33 Binhagi S, Chapot R, Rogopoulos A, Houdart E: Carotid stenting of chronic cervical dissection aneurysm: A report of two cases. Neurology 2002;59:935–937.
34 Butterworth RJ, Thomas DJ, Wolfe JHN, Mansfield AO, Al-Kutoubi A: Endovascular treatment of carotid dissecting aneurysms. Cerebrovasc Dis 1999;9:242–247.
35 Liu AY, Paulsen RD, Marcellus ML, Steinberg GK, Marks MP: Long-term outcomes after carotid stent placement for treatment of carotid artery dissection. Neurosurgery 1999;45:1368–1374.
36 Schievink WI: Spontaneous dissection of the carotid and vertebral arteries. N Engl J Med 2001;344:898–906.
37 Houser OW, Mokri B, Sundt TM Jr, Baker HL Jr, Reese DF: Spontaneous cervical cephalic arterial dissection and its residuum: Angiographic spectrum. AJNR Am J Neuroradiol 1984;5:27–34.
38 Steinke W, Rautenberg W, Schwartz A, Hennerici M: Noninvasive monitoring of internal carotid artery dissection. Stroke 1994;25:998–1005.
39 Pozzati E, Giuliani G, Acciarri N, Nuzzo G: Long-term follow-up of occlusive cervical carotid dissection. Stroke 1990;21:528–531.
40 Leclerc X, Lucas C, Godefroy O, Tessa H, Martinat P, Leys D, Pruvo JP: Helical CT for the follow-up of cervical internal carotid artery dissections. AJNR Am J Neuroradiol 1998;19:831–837.

41 Leclerc X, Lucas C, Godefroy O, Nicol L, Moretti A, Leys D, Pruvo JP: Preliminary experience using contrast-enhanced MR angiography to assess vertebral artery structure for the follow-up of suspected dissection. AJNR Am J Neuroradiol 1999;20:1482–1490.
42 Caso V, Paciaroni M, Corea F, Hamam M, Milia P, Pelliccioli GP, Parnetti L, Gallai V: Recanalization of cervical artery dissection: Influencing factors and role in neurological outcome. Cerebrovasc Dis 2004;17:93–97.
43 Youl BD, Coutellier A, Dubois B, Leger JM, Bousser MG: Three cases of spontaneous extracranial vertebral artery dissection. Stroke 1990;21:618–625.
44 Touze E, Oppenheim C, Zuber M, Meary E, Meder JF, Mas JL: Early asymptomatic recurrence of cervical artery dissection: Three cases. Neurology 2003;61:572–574.
45 Schievink WI, Michels VV, Piepgras DG: Neurovascular manifestations of heritable connective disorders: A review. Stroke 1994;25:889–903.
46 Schievink WI, Mokri B, Piepgras DG, Kuiper JD: Recurrent spontaneous arterial dissections: Risk in familial versus nonfamilial disease. Stroke 1996;27:622–624.
47 Schievink WI, Wijdicks EF, Michels VV, Vockley J, Godfrey M: Heritable connective tissue disorders in cervical artery dissections: A prospective study. Neurology 1998;50:1166–1169.
48 Hill MD, Hwa G, Perry JR: Extracranial cervical artery dissection. Stroke 2000;31:799.
49 Lucas C, Moulin T, Deplanque D, Tatu L, Chavot D: Stroke patterns of internal carotid artery dissection in 40 patients. Stroke 1998;29:2646–2648.
50 Engelter ST, Lyrer PA, Kirsch EC, Steck AJ: Long-term follow-up after extracranial internal carotid artery dissection. Eur Neurol 2000;44:199–204.

Dr. Emmanuel Touzé
Service de Neurologie, Hôpital Sainte-Anne
1 rue Cabanis
FR–75674 Paris Cedex 14 (France)
Tel. +33 1 45 65 88 58, Fax +33 1 45 65 87 94, E-Mail e.touze@ch-sainte-anne.fr

Baumgartner RW, Bogousslavsky J, Caso V, Paciaroni M (eds): Handbook on Cerebral Artery Dissection. Front Neurol Neurosci. Basel, Karger, 2005, vol 20, pp 140–146

Thrombolysis in Cervical Artery Dissection

Dimitrios Georgiadis, Ralf W. Baumgartner

Department of Neurology, University of Zürich, Zürich, Switzerland

Abstract

Safety and efficacy of intravenous (IVT) and intra-arterial thrombolysis (LIT) in patients with acute stroke due to spontaneous cervical artery dissection were not assessed in any controlled randomized trial. Data on IVT are derived from 4 studies with a total of 50 patients aged 48 ± 10 years with internal carotid artery dissection. No new or worsened local signs on the side of dissection, such as Horner syndrome and cranial nerve palsy, and no rupture of the cervical carotid artery or subarachnoid hemorrhage (SAH) were observed. One patient dramatically deteriorated during IVT, probably due to arterial embolism arising from a thrombus dislocated from the dissection site. Mortality was 8%, while 40% of patients had a good outcome defined by a modified Rankin scale (mRS) score of 0–2 points. Up to date, a total of 15 patients with carotid or vertebral artery dissection treated with LIT were described. No intracranial hemorrhage, rupture of the dissected vessel, SAH, or recurrent arterial embolism were reported in any patient. Mortality was 13%, while good outcome (mRS score 0–2 points) was observed in 60% of patients, which is comparable to the results in the active group of the PROACT II study. Currently available data thus suggest that IVT should not be withheld in patients with acute stroke due to cervical artery dissection. LIT treatment can only be based on individual decision-making.

Intravenous Thrombolysis

No randomized study has yet examined effectiveness or potential hazards of IVT or LIT thrombolysis in acute ischemic stroke caused by spontaneous internal carotid or vertebral artery dissection; currently available data on this issue are thus derived from small case series or case reports. In this chapter, safety and efficacy of IVT and LIT will be discussed.

Ischemic stroke caused by spontaneous internal carotid (sICAD) or vertebral artery dissection (sVAD) was not an exclusion criterion in any of the major thrombolysis trials; still, these patients were not specifically identified prior to treatment, or retrospectively analyzed as a subgroup. The presence of an intramural hematoma and intraluminal thrombus in the dissected vessel suggest that intravenous thrombolysis (IVT) may be associated with additional risks: axial and/or longitudinal extension of the vessel wall hematoma, causing (1) new or progressive local signs on the side of dissection, such as Horner syndrome and cranial nerve palsy; (2) progression of luminal narrowing; (3) pseudoaneurysm formation; (4) vessel rupture causing cervical or subarachnoid hemorrhage (SAH), and (5) arterial embolism through thrombus dislocation.

Up to date, a total of 50 patients (sICAD in all cases) were described in four observational studies [1–4], which are summarized in table 1. The dose of recombinant tissue plasminogen activator applied in one study was 0.8 mg/kg, while 10/11 patients were treated within the 3- to 6-hour window; 2 of 33 patients in another study received treatment 3–4.5 h after symptom onset, while remaining patients were treated according to the National Institute of Neurological Disorders and Stroke (NINDS) trial protocol [5]. The observations made are as follows:

(1) No new or progressing local signs were observed in any patient.

(2) Progression of luminal narrowing was hard to assess from the available data, particularly because only one study [1] examined patients both, before and after IVT, while patients were examined on a single occasion in remaining studies. Thus, the only information available can be derived from the degree of stenosis after IVT as compared to the natural history of the disease, and even this comparison is of limited value due to the low number of thrombolyzed patients and the lack of specific information concerning exact degree of stenosis and timing of follow-up vascular studies. Internal carotid artery (ICA) occlusion was present in 27 of 50 (54%) patients. ICA stenosis, the exact degree of which is not mentioned, was observed in 3 of 11 patients in one study [2], and ICA stenosis >50% in 8 of 33 patients in another [4]; data from a further study had to be excluded from this evaluation, as the authors merely described a stepwise recanalization, without providing actual information on the presence or degree of stenosis [1]. Thus, we can only conclude that ICA stenosis following IVT was present in 11 of 44 (25%) of patients. A recent study described cervical ICA occlusion or severe stenosis in 70% of 145 sICAD patients presenting with acute ischemic symptoms, who did not undergo IVT. Vascular findings were obtained using ultrasound examinations, which were performed a median of 2 days (range 0–114 days) after symptom onset [6]. While these findings appear comparable to the ones mentioned above, both, methodological issues and the small number of enrolled patients preclude any meaningful conclusions.

Table 1. Studies on intravenous thrombolysis in acute ischemic stroke caused by spontaneous dissection of the cervical internal carotid artery

Author	Patient	Cervical carotid artery findings after thrombolysis (time interval symptom onset or thrombolysis to vascular assessment)	New/worsened Horner syndrome or cranial nerve palsy on side of dissection; carotid rupture, cervical or SAH	Pseudoaneurysm of cervical carotid artery	Arterial embolism	Clinical outcome
Rudolf et al. [1]	6	Stepwise recanalization, n = 4 Persisting occlusion, n = 2 (Not reported)	0	0	0	NIHSS 0, n = 2; 1, 9, n = 2 mRS 0, n = 2; 2, 4, n = 2 Died, n = 2
Derex et al. [2]	11	Occlusion, n = 8; stenosis, n = 3[1] (8 ± 7 days after symptom onset)	0	1	0	mRS 0–1; n = 4; 3–4; n = 7
Georgiadis et al. [4]	33[2]	Normal, n = 8 Stenosis 50–70%, n = 2; ≥70%, n = 6 Occlusion, n = 17 (17–52 h after thrombolysis)	0	0	1	Median NIHSS, 7 (range, 5–9) mRS 0–2, n = 17; 3–5, n = 14 Died, n = 2

[1] All dissected cervical internal carotid arteries were initially occluded.
[2] Two patients described by Georgiadis et al. were already published by Arnold et al. [3].
mRS = Modified Rankin scale; NIHSS = National Institute of Health Stroke Scale.

(3) One pseudoaneurysm was observed in 44 patients who underwent MR or catheter angiography after IVT. Thus, one pseudoaneurysm was diagnosed in 19 (5.2%) nonoccluded sICAD (table 1). Pseudoaneurysms were reported to occur in 13–48% of patients with sICAD [7–10]. Thus, the present data do not suggest that IVT promotes the development of pseudoaneurysm in patients with sICAD.

(4) No patient showed clinical or radiological signs of cervical or SAH.

(5) A dramatic deterioration during IVT was observed in one patient by Georgiadis et al. [4], and attributed to arterial embolism, probably by a thrombus dislocated from the sICAD. Still, the authors could obviously provide no conclusive evidence to support this assumption. No deterioration attributable to IVT was reported in the other studies.

The low number of patients examined, and the fact that none of the above-mentioned studies were randomized, prohibits any conclusions concerning influence of IVT on outcome. Overall, mRS $\leq$2 was observed in 20 of 50 (40%) patients. These results are comparable to the ones reported in the NINDS trial (mRS $\leq$2 in 48% of cases) [5]; still, it must be taken into account, that sICAD patients were younger (48 $\pm$ 10 vs. 69 $\pm$ 12 years, respectively; mean $\pm$ SD), with slightly higher stroke severity (median 16 vs. 14, respectively; note that no NIHSS data were provided by Derex et al. [2]). Mortality was 8%, as compared to the 17.3% reported in the NINDS trial [5].

The aforementioned preliminary data suggest that IVT in patients with sICAD is not per se associated with additional risks or worse functional outcome as compared to patients with acute ischemic stroke of other etiologies. Therefore, it appears justified to apply IVT in sICAD patients. Safety and efficacy of this approach though, can only be evaluated through a prospective randomized study.

Local Intra-Arterial Thrombolysis

The possible complications of local intra-arterial thrombolysis (LIT) include those mentioned for IVT, but also the risk of catheter angiography and in particular thromboembolism due to the passage of the catheter through the occluded or severely narrowed dissected vessel and the catheterization of the false lumen. An overview of the published data is presented in table 2. Except for one study, describing 7 patients [3], remaining publications consist of reports including 1–2 cases [11–17]. No rupture of the dissected vessel, cervical or SAH, or intracranial hemorrhage, or peri-interventional arterial embolism was reported in any study. Thus, based on the currently available, albeit limited data, LIT in acute ischemic stroke due to sICAD or sVAD is not

Table 2. Studies on local intra-arterial thrombolysis in acute ischemic stroke caused by spontaneous dissection of the cervical internal carotid artery

Study	N/Age/Sex	Dissected vessel	Time from symptom onset to thrombolysis, min (drug)	New/worsened Horner syndrome or cranial nerve palsy on side of dissection; carotid rupture; cervical or SAH; cervical pseudoaneurysm	Clinical outcome, mRS (time after thrombolysis)
Price et al. [11]	1/33/M	VA	? (rtPA)	0	1 (6 months)
Sampognaro et al. [12]	1/38/M	ICA	170 (UK)	0	0 (6 months)
Ahmad et al. [13]	1/28/F	VA bi	? (UK)	0	died (5 days)
	2/41/F	VA	? (UK)	0	1 (?)
Arnold et al. [3]	1/40 /F	VA bi	80 (UK)	0	1 (3 months)
	2/48/F	ICA	175 (UK)	0	1 (3 months)
	3/40/F	ICA	250 (UK)	0	3 (3 months)
	4/68/M	VA	210 (UK)	0	1 (3 months)
	5/43/F	VA	385 (UK)	0	died (3 months)
	6/43/M	VA bi	285 (UK)	0	5 (3 months)
	7/52/M	ICA	225 (UK)	0	4 (3 months)
Restrepo et al. [15]	1/34/F	VA	2,580 (rtPA)	0	1 (6 months)
Ogiwara et al. [16]	1/22/M	ICA	120 (UK)	0	0 (8 months)
Abboud et al. [17]	1/44/M	ICA	210 (UK)	0	0 (7 days)

bi = Bilateral; ICA = internal carotid artery; min = minutes; rtPA = recombinant tissue plasminogen activator; UK = urokinase; VA = vertebral artery.

associated with any additional risks. Assessment of treatment efficacy is also hampered by the marked variation in severity of initial neurological deficit. Mortality was 13%, while good outcome (mRS ≤2) was observed in 60% of patients. These results compare favorably to the ones reported in the Intra-Arterial Prourokinase for Acute Ischemic Stroke (PROACT) II study (mortality 25%; mRS ≤2 in 40% of patients) [18]. Still, two obvious differences must be noted: (1) patients with acute ischemic stroke caused by sICAD or sVAD were notably younger as compared to PROACT II patients (41 ± 11 and 64 ± 10 years, respectively, mean ± SD) and (2) only patients with occlusion of the M1 or M2 segment of the middle cerebral artery were enrolled in PROACT II, while vertebrobasilar system lesions were present in 53% of patients with symptomatic cervical artery dissection treated with LIT.

The presented data do not allow any definitive statements or treatment recommendations regarding application of LIT in patients with sICAD or sVAD. We suggest that treatment can only be based on individual decision making, taking patients age, severity of clinical symptoms, and vascular status and accessibility of the occluded vessel for LIT into account.

References

1 Rudolf J, Neveling M, Grond M, Schmulling S, Stenzel C, Heiss W: Stroke following internal carotid artery occlusion – A contra-indication for intravenous thrombolysis? Eur J Neurol 1999;6: 51–55.

2 Derex L, Nighoghossian N, Turjman F, Hermier M, Honnorat J, Neuschwander P, Froment JC, Trouillas P: Intravenous tPA in acute ischemic stroke related to internal carotid artery dissection. Neurology 2000;54:2159–2161.

3 Arnold M, Nedeltchev K, Sturzenegger M, Schroth G, Loher TJ, Stepper F, Remonda L, Bassetti C, Mattle HP: Thrombolysis in patients with acute stroke caused by cervical artery dissection: Analysis of 9 patients and review of the literature. Arch Neurol 2002;59:549–553.

4 Georgiadis D, Schwab S, Engelter S, Roman Sztajzel R, Arnold M, Siebler M, Lyrer P, Baumgartner RW: Intravenous thrombolysis in patients with acute stroke due to spontaneous carotid dissection. Neurology 2005;64:1612–1614.

5 The National Institute of Neurological Disorders and Stroke rt-PA Study Group: Tissue plasminogen activator for acute ischemic stroke. N Engl J Med 1995;333:1581–1587.

6 Baumgartner RW, Arnold M, Baumgartner I, Mosso M, Gönner F, Studer A, Schroth G, Schuknecht B, Sturzenegger M: Carotid dissection with and without ischemic events: local symptoms and cerebral artery findings. Neurology 2001;57:827–832.

7 Houser OW, Mokri B, Sundt TMJ, Baker HL, Reese DF: Spontaneous cervical cephalic arterial dissection and its residuum: Angiographic spectrum. AJNR Am J Neuroradiol 1984;5:27–34.

8 Mokri B, Sundt TMJ, Houser OW, Piepgras DW: Spontaneous dissection of the cervical internal carotid artery. Ann Neurol 1986;19:126–138.

9 Ast G, Woimant F, Georges B, Laurian C, Haguenau M: Spontaneous dissection of the internal carotid artery in 68 patients. Eur J Med 1993;2:466–472.

10 Guillon B, Brunerau L, Biousse V, Djouhri H, Lévy C, Bousser MG: Long-term follow-up of aneurysms developed during extracranial internal carotid artery dissection. Neurology 1999;53: 117–122.

11 Price RF, Sellar R, Leung C, O'Sullivan MJ: Traumatic vertebral arterial dissection and vertebrobasilar thrombosis successfully treated with endovascular thrombolysis and stenting. AJNR Am J Neuroradiol 1998;19:1677–1680.

12 Sampognaro G, Turgut T, Conners J Jr, White C, Collins T, Ramee SR: Intra-arterial thrombolysis in a patient presenting with an ischemic stroke due to spontaneous internal carotid artery dissection. Catheter Cardiovasc Interv 1999;48:312–315.

13 Ahmad HA, Gerraty RP, Davis SM, Cameron PA: Cervicocerebral artery dissections. J Accid Emerg Med 1999;16:422–424.

14 Zaidat OO, Fernandes Filho JA, Singh G, Suarez JI: Thrombolytic therapy for acute extra-cranial artery dissection: Report of two cases. Arq Neuropsiquiatr 2001;59:936–938.

15 Restrepo L, Pradilla G, Llinas R, Beauchamp NJ: Perfusion- and diffusion-weighted MR imaging-guided therapy of vertebral artery dissection: Intraarterial thrombolysis through an occipital vertebral anastomosis. AJNR Am J Neuroradiol 2003;24:1823–1826.

16 Ogiwara H, Maeda K, Hara T, Kimura T, Abe H: Spontaneous intracranial internal carotid artery dissection treated by intra-arterial thrombolysis and superficial temporal artery-middle cerebral artery anastomosis in the acute stage – Case report. Neurol Med Chir (Tokyo) 2005;45:148–151.

17 Abboud H, Houdart E, Meseguer E, Amarenco P: Stent assisted endovascular thrombolysis of internal carotid artery dissection. J Neurol Neurosurg Psychiatry 2005;76:292–293.

18 Furlan A, Higashida R, Wechsler L, Gent M, Rowley H, Kase C, Pessin M, Ahuja A, Callahan F, Clark WM, Silver F, Rivera F, for the PROACT Investigators: Intra-arterial prourokinase for acute ischemic stroke. The PROACT II study: A randomized controlled trial. JAMA 1999;282: 2003–2011.

PD Dr. Dimitrios Georgiadis
Department of Neurology, University Hospital
Frauenklinikstrasse 26, CH–8091 Zürich (Switzerland)
Tel. +41 1 255 5565, Fax +41 1 255 8864
E-Mail dimitrios.georgiadis@usz.ch

Baumgartner RW, Bogousslavsky J, Caso V, Paciaroni M (eds): Handbook on Cerebral Artery Dissection. Front Neurol Neurosci. Basel, Karger, 2005, vol 20, pp 147–159

Antithrombotic Therapy for Cervical Artery Dissection

S. Engelter, P. Lyrer

Neurological Clinic and Stroke Unit, University Hospital Basel, Basel, Switzerland

Abstract

Antithrombotic therapy in patients with cervical artery dissection (CAD) is empiric rather than evidence based. The routine use of anticoagulants in each CAD patient cannot be recommended. A randomized controlled trial comparing antiplatelets with anticoagulation is clearly needed. However, due to the large sample size, which is required to gather meaningful results, such a trial is a huge venture. Thus, the matter of antithrombotic treatment in CAD is not expected to be solved in the near future. What should clinicians do in the meantime? There are several pathophysiological arguments in favor as well as against anticoagulants or antiplatelets. Until more data are available, it is our personal recommendation that treatment decisions should be geared to several clinical and paraclinical features of individual patients. The chapter compiles putative arguments in favor versus against immediate anticoagulation and may be helpful for individually tailored antithrombotic treatment decisions in CAD patients.

Cervical artery dissection (CAD) was first recognized as a cause of ischemic stroke in the mid 1950s [1, 2] although there are pathological reports on the condition dating from 1872 [3]. The incidence of cervical internal carotid artery dissection (ICAD) is about 2–3/100,000 per year [4, 5]. For cervical vertebral artery dissection (VAD) community-based epidemiological data are absent. Based on hospital-based case series, VAD incidence is estimated to be about 1–1.5 per 100,000 per year [6]. The recurrence rate of stroke in CAD is less than 1% per year [7–10], except for familial cases. Although anticoagulation is recommended by many authors [11–13], there is no reliable evidence from randomized trials of the efficacy of this therapy [6, 14–16].

In this therapeutic dilemma, physicians still face CAD patients for two main therapeutic goals. First, to prevent stroke, recurrent stroke or other disabling complications. Second, to provide optimal conditions for rehabilitation in order to facilitate functional recovery in those who already had a stroke due to CAD. The latter issue, however, is not the subject of this chapter. Our objective is to provide an overview about the pathophysiology and clinical experience with anticoagulation as well as antiplatelets in CAD patients. Specifically, we discuss pathophysiological considerations in favor as well as against anticoagulation. Thereafter, we present a systematic meta-analysis of the existing clinical data on antithrombotic therapy in ICAD.

Pathophysiological Arguments in Favor of Anticoagulation in CAD

CAD occurs when blood penetrates through a subintimal tear into the arterial wall leading to intramural hematoma. Mural hematoma results in arterial narrowing causing stenosis or vessel occlusion. Stroke in CAD is either a consequence of embolism originating from the injured intima or from hemodynamic compromise. Blood accumulation can also occur subadventitially, which may result in local compression syndromes or in subarachnoidal hemorrhage, which occurs more often in intracranial than in extracranial dissections.

Transcranial Doppler sonography monitoring studies revealed microembolic signals downstream of the dissected arteries. In ICAD, high-intensity transient signals (HITS) suggesting embolism were detected in the middle cerebral artery. In VAD, HITS were shown in the posterior cerebral artery [17]. The frequency of HITS in CAD patients is reported within the range of 25–60% [17–21]. However, sample sizes of 6–28 patients limit the significance of these numbers. HITS seem to occur more often among those CAD patients who present with stroke compared to those with nonischemic signs and symptoms [18]. Most CAD patients with recurrent ischemia had HITS (i.e. 6/7 [20], and 3/3 [17], respectively). These observations may indicate that CAD patients with HITS have an increased stroke risk due to assumed embolism and require stronger antithrombotic therapy. However, HITS occur despite antithrombotic therapy, too [17, 21]. Furthermore, no association was recorded between the presence or number of HITS and the type of antithrombotic treatment (i.e. anticoagulants or -platelets) [21]. Among a population of 20 CAD patients, all 5 HITS-positive ones had some form of antithrombotic therapy during transcranial Doppler sonography monitoring. This was heparin in 3, aspirin in one, and aspirin plus heparin in another patient, respectively [17].

Conventional angiography studies in ICAD patients visualized occlusions of branches of the anterior or middle cerebral arteries in several patients [22–24]. The frequency of this angiographic finding has been reported within a range of 14% (3/19) [23], 16% (5/36) [22], and even 50% (4/8) [24]. Positive findings of distal branch occlusions or microemboli are strong arguments in favor of an embolic pathomechanism in stroke due to CAD.

Analyses of the infarct lesion pattern on CT or T2-weighted magnetic resonance imaging in ICAD-stroke patients revealed that the vast majority had cortical, large subcortical or mixed cortical-subcortical lesions. Only 3–16% had borderzone lesions according to most studies [25–28]. Similar findings were reported in a mixed population of ICAD and VAD [29]. Only one group reported contrary results with nearly 50% borderzone infarcts [30]. More recently, diffusion-weighted magnetic resonance imaging, revealed that 10 out of 14 (71%) ICAD patients had multiple diffusion-weighted magnetic resonance imaging lesions [31]. These findings suggested that in most patients, artery-to-artery embolism rather than hemodynamic compromise is the main underlying mechanism in stroke due to ICAD.

In summary, the evidence of microembolic ultrasound signals, distal branch emboli in angiography, and the results of studies on infarct topography, seem to point towards embolism as the crucial stroke mechanism in the majority of CAD patients. In analogy to cardioembolic stroke (e.g. atrial fibrillation), where anticoagulation is superior to antiplatelets (e.g. aspirin) in respect of secondary stroke prevention, these observations would favor anticoagulation in stroke prevention of CAD.

Another, at least theoretical, argument in favor of anticoagulation is the risk of clot formation in cases of arterial occlusion due to CAD. Cases with free-floating thrombi in dissected internal carotid arteries (ICAs) have indeed been reported occasionally [32, 33]. In addition, most occluded arteries recanalize over time; 30% within 8 days and 60–80% within 3 months [34, 35]. During the recanalization process, clots may be mobilized and transported downstream, where they can cause blockage of intracranial arteries prompting embolic infarctions [36].

Pathophysiological Arguments against Anticoagulation in CAD

CAD means intramural bleeding. At least theoretically, anticoagulation may lead to enlargement of the mural bleed, because heparin or warfarin inhibits coagulation. In case of anticoagulation-mediated perpetuation or recurrence of intramural bleeding, increase of the outer vessel diameter may cause local compression symptoms, such as painful Horner's syndrome or cranial nerve palsies. More important, hemodynamic worsening can occur, which implies the risk of low-flow infarcts of supplied brain tissue. Delayed occlusion of the ICA during heparin therapy was indeed recently reported in 5 out of 20 patients with ICAD [37]. The activated partial thromboplastin time ratio was significantly higher in patients with delayed ICA occlusion (2.6 ± 0.4) versus those without (2.0 ± 0.5) [37]. Thus, the likelihood for delayed ICA occlusion seems to increase with higher degrees of anticoagulation. Although the direct evidence of an extended mural hematoma was lacking, it was speculated that (relative) overshooting anticoagulation might have caused mural rebleeding, which caused ongoing lumen narrowing until complete ICA occlusion. Whether the relationship between anticoagulation and delayed carotid occlusion is really causal rather than coincidental requires further studies. In 4 of these 5 ICAD patients delayed ICA occlusion during i.v. heparin occurred clinically silent. However, one of these 5 patients developed a watershed infarct. He was the only one with an unfavorable collateralization at the Circle of Willis, suggesting a hemodynamic stroke mechanism. In the majority of patients, delayed loss of arterial patency was not associated with clinical worsening. However, whether delayed heparin-associated carotid occlusion led to a delay in stroke recovery remains an open question. These observations show that anticoagulants may cause harm in some individual CAD patients.

In addition, a recent meta-analysis showed that for acute stroke patients in general, immediate anticoagulation had neither short- nor long-term benefit [38].

Clinical Experience with Antiplatelets and Anticoagulation in CAD

Some patients with stroke due to CAD report preceding warning symptoms mostly within a week before the index stroke [39, 40]. This observation implies that there might be a chance to prevent stroke in such patients. However, this optimistic view is clouded by the fact that in half of these patients the interval between inaugural symptoms and stroke is only in the magnitude of minutes to hours [40].

In VAD, there are single case reports about subarachnoid hemorrhage as the presenting feature [41, 42], in which antithrombotic treatment and particularly anticoagulation is considered deleterious. However, this feature is unusual and should prompt the search for an accompanying intracranial dissection. The latter leads to subarachnoid hemorrhage in more than 20% [29].

Stroke occurrence or recurrence has been reported in ICAD patients treated with antiplatelets [12], as well as in those with sufficient anticoagulation [34, 43–45], indicating that the avoidance of first or further strokes even with anticoagulation is not granted.

In one recent case series of more than 100 CAD patients, stroke during follow-up was recorded in neither treatment group. However, recurrent transient ischemic attacks occurred in only 1 out of 113 CAD patients with anticoagulation, compared to 6 out of 9 patients with antiplatelets. In turn, one

Table 1. Dichotomized outcome assessment based on information extractable from publications: criteria for 'no or minor disability' versus 'major disability' [15]

Where modified Rankin Scale (mRS) [47] is reported, mRS 0–2 are judged as 'no or minor disability', mRS 3–5 'major disability'.

Patients who are reported to be able to return to their original or similar job (part/fulltime) were classified as having 'no disability'.

Patients described as 'mild/slight or no deficits', 'asymptomatic' or 'markedly improved' were also classified as 'no or minor disability'.

Patients described as 'improved' (without further detailed information) were classified as 'major disability', as were patients with 'persisting neurological deficits such as hemiparesis'. Patients who had to be transferred to a nursing home or who needed permanent help for daily living were also classified in the 'major disability' group.

---

anticoagulated patient suffered from symptomatic intracerebral hemorrhage, while none of the patients with antiplatelets did so [40]. These findings illustrate the need to balance risk and benefits of either agent in a comprehensive way. Even in the absence of randomized controlled trials, a systematic meta-analysis of the available data can provide clinically useful information about the effects in CAD patients treated either with anticoagulants or with antiplatelets.

Systematic Meta-Analysis about Antithrombotic Drugs for ICAD

The systematic meta-analysis aimed, first, to determine whether antithrombotic drugs (antiplatelet drugs, anticoagulation) are effective and safe in the treatment of patients with ICAD and, second, which is the better treatment. The challenge was to perform a systemic meta-analysis in order to gather the best available evidence for antithrombotic treatment in ICAD without any controlled trials on this matter although these are usually the base of Cochrane Reviews [15]. The authors sought after nonrandomized studies with ≥4 patients, which reported on outcomes with stratification to the used type of antithrombotic therapy (i.e., anticoagulation, antiplatelets, or neither). Antiplatelets mean acetylsalicylic acid, ticlopidine, clopidogrel, sulfinpyrazone, and dipyridamole. Anticoagulation means full-dose anticoagulants, such as i.v. or s.c. fractionated or unfractionated heparin or oral coumarin. The first choice treatment was taken for analyses ('intention-to-treat' approach).

Predefined primary outcomes were 'dead from all causes' and 'dead or disabled' at the end of the follow-up period (criteria for disability are shown on table 1). The authors intended to specify the length of follow-up after which outcome assessment should take place (e.g. 3 months). The lack of such information made it necessary to use the latest outcome evaluation extractable from the studies. Due to the lack of data it was also not possible to attribute each death as stroke-related, related to other vascular disease, or from nonvascular causes. Secondary outcomes were first stroke occurrence, stroke recurrence, any stroke during reported follow-up, extra- and intracranial hemorrhage. Data on primary and secondary outcomes were extracted independently by two raters. Disagreements were resolved by discussion. The authors used as data sources first the Cochrane Stroke Group specialized Trials Register. Second, comprehensive searches of MEDLINE (1966 – May 2002) and EMBASE (1980 – June 2002) were done. Third, reference lists of all relevant papers were checked for additional eligible studies.

No reliable comparisons of antiplatelets or -coagulants with control (i.e. 'no antithrombotic treatment') were available. For comparative analyses of both agents, 26 studies including 327 patients (who either received antiplatelet drugs or anticoagulants) were eligible. Two of one hundred and nine patients (1.8%) treated with antiplatelets were reported dead, and 4 of 218 (1.8%) treated with anticoagulants, respectively. The weighted estimates across studies show that the likelihood of death within the follow-up period does not differ between both treatment groups as indicated by a Peto odds ratio of 1.59, with a 95% confidence interval (CI) 0.22–11.59. Details are shown in figure 1.

Due to the lack of data, the analysis in respect of the outcome 'dead or disabled' was based on fewer (i.e. 20) studies. Fourteen of fifty-nine patients (23.7%) treated with antiplatelets were dead or disabled, whereas 17 of 119 (14.3%) patients treated with anticoagulants met the criteria. These discrepant frequencies, which are based on accumulated events irrespectively of the studies they were derived from, seem to indicate a trend in favor of anticoagulants. However, the weighted estimate across all studies reveals that such an impression was misleading. The Peto odds ratio of 1.94 with a wide 95% CI of 0.76–4.91 clarifies that there is no significant difference in the odds of being 'dead or disabled' among both treatments groups. Details are shown in figure 2.

According to this systematic review of all relevant observational case studies, the frequency of death or poor outcome after ICAD seems to be low and lower than previously suggested.

Surprisingly, and in contrast to several treatment recommendations [11–13], there was no evidence that antiplatelets are less effective than anticoagulants in preventing stroke in ICAD patients. However, studies were sparse and showed conflicting findings. Only in five studies strokes under antithrombotic therapy were reported with details on the applied therapy. While in one study stroke occurred in 6 out of 8 patients with antiplatelets, other studies did not report similar observations, but reported stroke under anticoagulation in 3–16% of their patients. Three out of ninety-one patients (3.3%) with 'no

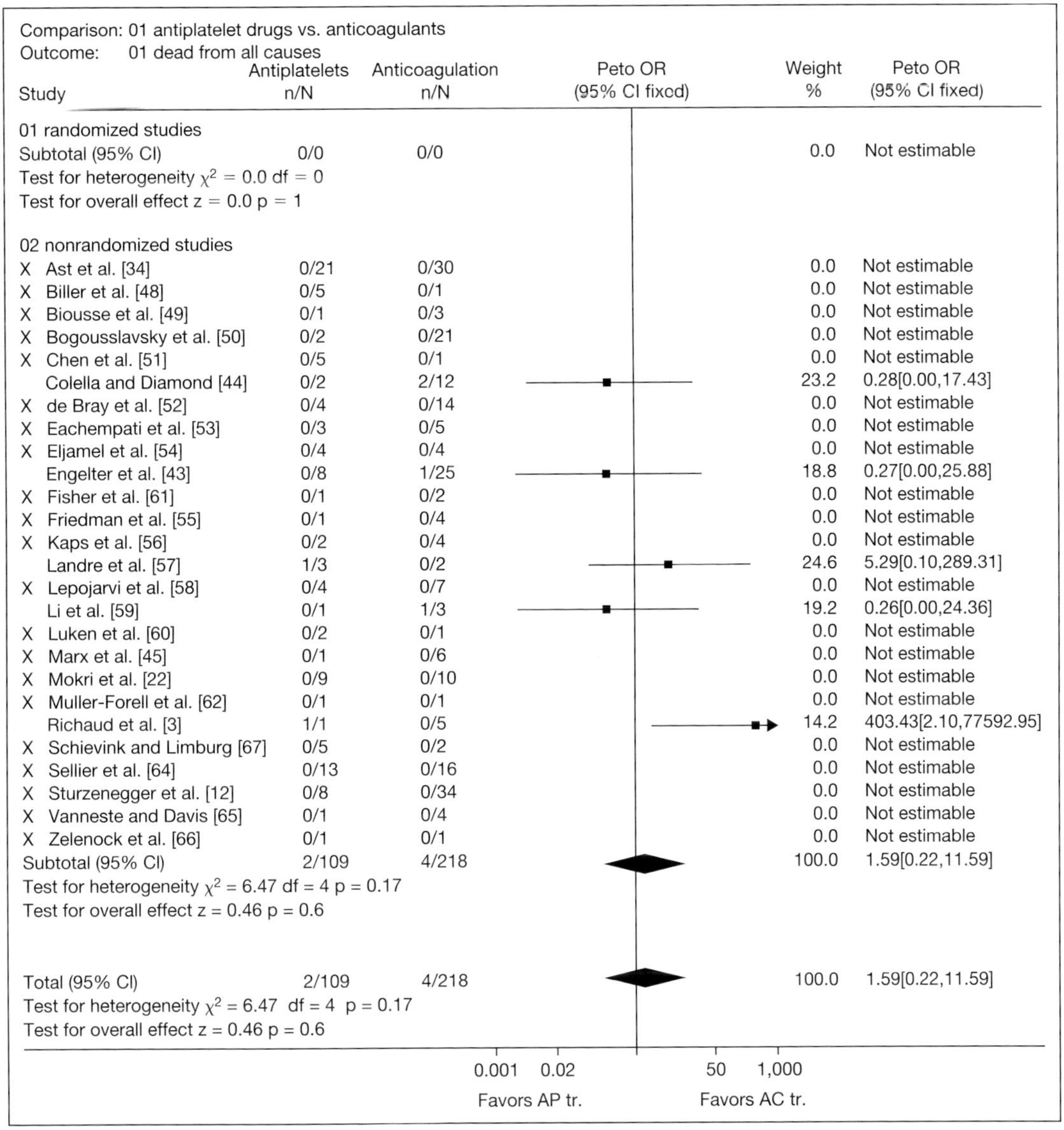

Fig. 1. Likelihood for 'dead from all causes' among ICAD patients treated with anticoagulation compared to those with antiplatelets. Results are expressed as Peto odds ratio (OR) with a fixed-effects model. OR > 1 suggest anticoagulants to be superior to antiplatelets [15]. (Reproduced with permission from John Wiley & Sons Ltd.). Modified from [16] (with permission of the American Heart Association, Inc©). Included studies were case series with ≥4 patients which reported on the outcome 'dead from all causes' at the end of follow-up with stratification to the used type of antithrombotic therapy (i.e. anticoagulation or antiplatelets) [3, 12, 22, 44–46, 48–64].

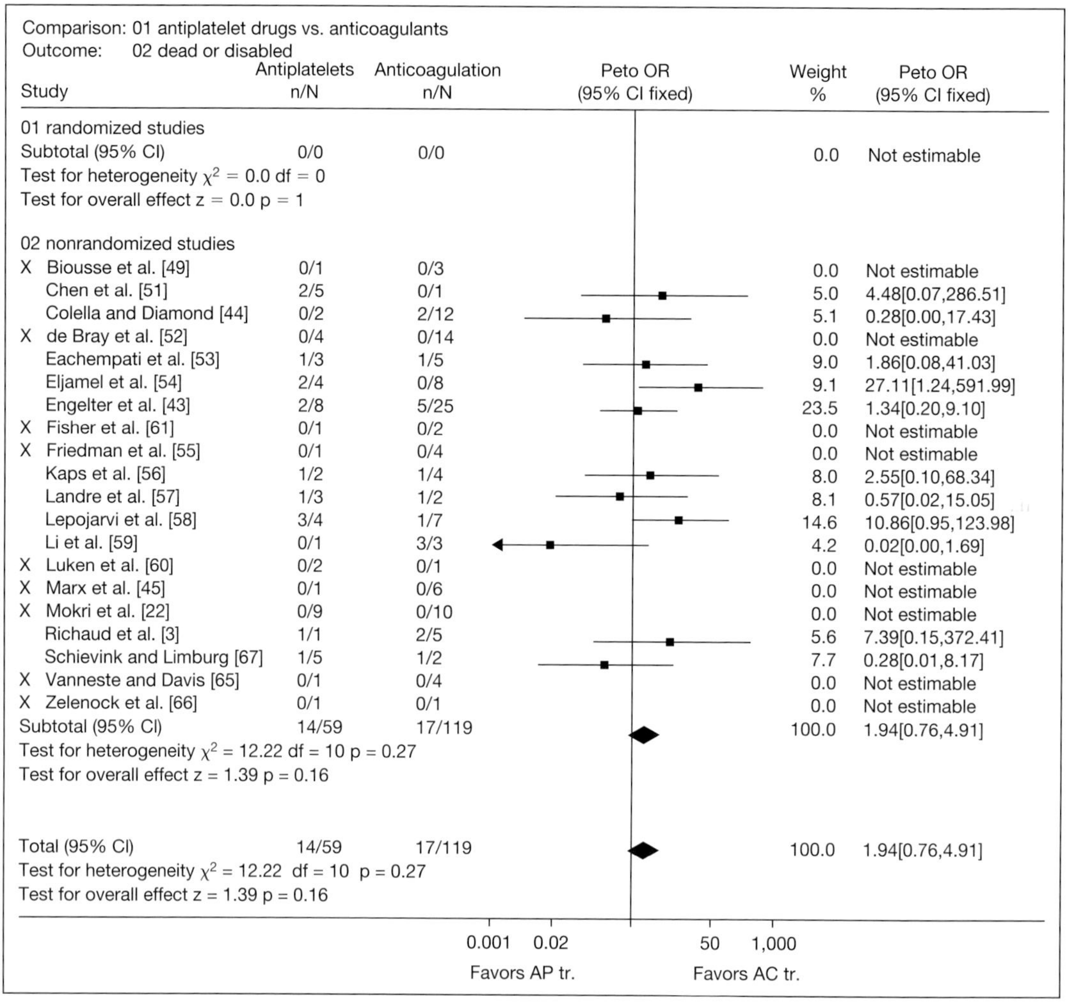

Fig. 2. Likelihood for 'dead or disabled' among ICAD patients treated with anticoagulation versus antiplatelets. Results are expressed as Peto odds ratio (OR) with a fixed-effects model. OR >1 suggest anticoagulants to be superior to antiplatelets [15]. (Reproduced with permission from John Wiley & Sons Ltd.). Modified from [16] (with permission of the American Heart Association, Inc©). Included studies were case series with ≥4 patients which reported on the outcome 'dead or disabled' at the end of follow-up with stratification to the used type of antithrombotic therapy (i.e. anticoagulation or antiplatelets) [3, 22, 43–45, 49, 51–61, 65–67].

Table 2. Clinical and paraclinical features as putative arguments in favor or against immediate anticoagulation in individual CAD patients at the time of diagnosis

Feature	In favor of immediate anticoagulation	Against immediate anticoagulation	Comment/references
Severe strokes (i.e. NIHSSS ≥15)		+	In analogy to findings of increased rate of symptomatic hemorrhagic transformation in severe strokes in TOAST [68]. Applying general ASA guidelines for anticoagulation [69].
Brain-imaging study not available		+	CAD can present with bleeds [41, 42]. Applying general ASA guidelines for anticoagulation [69].
Insufficient intracranial collaterals		+	Watershed infarct in patient without collaterals and with delayed ICA occlusion under heparin [37]. Single case.
Accompanying intracranial dissection, e.g. vertebral artery		+	Bleeding risk ↑ in intracranial dissection [29].
Local compression syndromes without stroke/TIA		+	
HITS	+		HITS more frequent in patients with recurrent ischemia [17, 20]. Few studies. HITS surrogate marker of 'microclots'?
Distal branch occlusions	+		Assumed correlative of distal embolism. Requires conventional angiography [22, 23].
Occlusion/ pseudoocclusion	+		Embolization may occur during recanalization [36].
Multiple TIAs/strokes affecting multiple regions of same circulation	+		Clinic may suggest repetitive emboli
Free-floating thrombus	+		Rare finding, requires conventional angiography [32, 33].

In the absence of evidence-based treatment guidelines, this synopsis is based on pathophysiological considerations, observations, and conclusions by analogy and reflects the view of the authors. Neither clinical/paraclinical features nor the comments/references claim to be exhaustive.

NIHSSS = National Institute of Health Stroke Scale Score; HITS = high-intensity transient signals; TIA = transient ischemic attacks; ICA = internal carotid artery; TOAST = Trial of Org 10172 in Acute Stroke Therapy; ASA = American Stroke Association.

antithrombotic therapy' had a first or recurrent stroke. Although this percentage is higher than for patients treated with antiplatelets (1.8%) or anticoagulants (1.8%), it does not necessarily reflect the assumed benefits of antithrombotic treatment. The differences may as well reflect a bias, such as that 'no antithrombotic treatment' could have been primarily applied to patients considered to have a bad prognosis. The same caution should be used in the interpretation of the observation that ICAD patients with surgery appeared to have a higher rate of death (6–11%), compared with those who received antithrombotic drugs (each 1.8%). This could be due to either treatment benefit of antithrombotic agents, or to selection bias (patients who were operated on were initially in a more serious stage of the disease), or to the surgery itself.

Intracranial bleeding is the major concern in antithrombotic treatment [38]. In ICAD, this risk seems to be low but possibly higher with anticoagulants than with antiplatelets based on the fact that 2 out of 414 (0.5%) patients on anticoagulation had intracranial hemorrhages, while none out of 157 patients with antiplatelets had the same complication [15]. However, nonrandomized studies are known to be highly susceptible to bias and outcome events may be under-represented [46].

As a consequence of these data, a large randomized controlled trial comparing anticoagulants and antiplatelets is desirable and ethically justified. Its protocol should include a stringent definition of carotid artery dissection, a standardized diagnostic protocol, strictly random allocation to different types of antithrombotic treatment, as well as accurate unbiased assessment of outcome. On the basis of the presented data we estimate a sample size of at least 1,200 patients in each treatment arm in order to detect a 5% difference in the proportion of patients dead or disabled from 20 to 15% (a 25% relative odds reduction).

Table 2 summarizes putative arguments in favor or against immediate anticoagulation of CAD patients.

References

1 Jentzer A: Dissecting aneurysm of the left internal carotid artery. Angiology 1954;5:232–234.

2 Anderson RM, Schechter MM: A case of spontaneous dissecting aneurysm of the internal carotid artery. J Neurol Neurosurg Psychiatry 1959;22:195–201.

3 Richaud J, Lagarrigue J, Lazorthes Y: [Traumatic injury affecting the extracranial portion of internal carotid artery (17 case reports)]. Neurochirurgie 1980;26:109–121.

4 Schievink WI, Mokri B, Whisnant JP: Internal carotid artery dissection in a community. Rochester, Minnesota, 1987–1992. Stroke 1993;24:1678–1680.

5 Giroud M, Fayolle H, Andre N, Dumas R, Becker F, Martin D, Baudoin N, Krause D: Incidence of internal carotid artery dissection in the community of Dijon. J Neurol Neurosurg Psychiatry 1994;57:1443.

6 Schievink WI: Spontaneous dissection of the carotid and vertebral arteries. N Engl J Med 2001;344:898–906.

7 Touze E, Gauvrit JY, Moulin T, Meder JF, Bracard S, Mas JL: Risk of stroke and recurrent dissection after a cervical artery dissection: A multicenter study. Neurology 2003;61:1347–1351.
8 Schievink WI, Mokri B, Piepgras DG: Spontaneous dissections of cervicocephalic arteries in childhood and adolescence. Neurology 1994;44:1607–1612.
9 Leys D, Moulin T, Stoikovic T, Begey S, Chavot D, DONALD Investigators: Follow up of patients with history of cervical artery dissection. Cerebrovasc Dis 1995;5:43–49.
10 Bassetti C, Carruzzo A, Sturzenegger M, Tuncdogan E: Recurrence of cervical artery dissection. A prospective study of 81 patients. Stroke 1996;27:1804–1807.
11 Hart RG, Easton JD: Dissections of cervical and cerebral arteries. Neurol Clin 1983;1:155–182.
12 Sturzenegger M: Spontaneous internal carotid artery dissection: Early diagnosis and management in 44 patients. J Neurol 1995;242:231–238.
13 Cimini N, D'Andrea P, Gentile M, Berletti R, Ferracci F, Candeago RM, Conte F, Moretto G: Cervical artery dissection: A 5-year prospective study in the Belluno district. Eur Neurol 2004;52:207–210.
14 Leys D, Lucas C, Gobert M, Deklunder G, Pruvo JP: Cervical artery dissections. Eur Neurol 1997;37:3–12.
15 Lyrer P, Engelter S: Antithrombotic drugs for carotid artery dissection. Cochrane Database Syst Rev 2003;(3):CD000255.
16 Lyrer P, Engelter S: Antithrombotic drugs for carotid artery dissection. Stroke 2004;35:613–614.
17 Droste DW, Junker K, Stogbauer F, Lowens S, Besselmann M, Braun B, et al: Clinically silent circulating microemboli in 20 patients with carotid or vertebral artery dissection. Cerebrovasc Dis 2001;12:181–185.
18 Srinivasan J, Newell DW, Sturzenegger M, Mayberg MR, Winn HR: Transcranial Doppler in the evaluation of internal carotid artery dissection. Stroke 1996;27:1226–1230.
19 Koennecke HC, Trocio SH Jr, Mast H, Mohr JP: Microemboli on transcranial Doppler in patients with spontaneous carotid artery dissection. J Neuroimaging 1997;7:217–220.
20 Molina CA, Alvarez-Sabin J, Schonewille W, Montaner J, Rovira A, Abilleira S, Codina A: Cerebral microembolism in acute spontaneous internal carotid artery dissection. Neurology 2000;55:1738–1740.
21 Oliveira V, Batista P, Soares F, Ferro JM: HITS in internal carotid dissections. Cerebrovasc Dis 2001;11:330–334.
22 Mokri B, Sundt TM Jr, Houser OW, Piepgras DG: Spontaneous dissection of the cervical internal carotid artery. Ann Neurol 1986;19:126–138.
23 Ehrenfeld WK, Wylie EJ: Spontaneous dissection of the internal carotid artery. Arch Surg 1976;111:1294–1301.
24 Petro GR, Witwer GA, Cacayorin ED, Hodge CJ, Bredenberg CE, Jastremski MS, Kieffer SA: Spontaneous dissection of the cervical internal carotid artery: Correlation of arteriography, CT, and pathology. AJR Am J Roentgenol 1987;148:393–398.
25 Steinke W, Schwartz A, Hennerici M: Topography of cerebral infarction associated with carotid artery dissection. J Neurol 1996;243:323–328.
26 Lucas C, Moulin T, Deplanque D, Tatu L, Chavot D: Stroke patterns of internal carotid artery dissection in 40 patients. Stroke 1998;29:2646–2648.
27 Milhaud D, de Freitas GR, van Melle G, Bogousslavsky J: Occlusion due to carotid artery dissection: A more severe disease than previously suggested. Arch Neurol 2002;59:557–561.
28 Benninger DH, Georgiadis D, Kremer C, Studer A, Nedeltchev K, Baumgartner RW: Mechanism of ischemic infarct in spontaneous carotid dissection. Stroke 2004;35:482–485.
29 Pelkonen O, Tikkakoski T, Pyhtinen J, Sotaniemi K: Cerebral CT and MRI findings in cervicocephalic artery dissection. Acta Radiol 2004;45:259–265.
30 Weiller C, Mullges W, Ringelstein EB, Buell U, Reiche W: Patterns of brain infarctions in internal carotid artery dissections. Neurosurg Rev 1991;14:111–113.
31 Koch S, Rabinstein AA, Romano JG, Forteza A: Diffusion-weighted magnetic resonance imaging in internal carotid artery dissection. Arch Neurol 2004;61:510–512.
32 Combe J, Poinsard P, Besancenot J, Camelot G, Cattin F, Bonneville JF, Moulin T, Henlin JL, Chopard JL, Cotte L: Free-floating thrombus of the extracranial internal carotid artery. Ann Vasc Surg 1990;4:558–562.

33 Cardon A, Aesch B, Mugnier B, Lucas A, Kerdiles Y: [Role of surgery in the treatment of dissections of the extracranial internal carotid artery. Apropos of a case, review of the literature]. J Chir (Paris) 1992;129:324–326.
34 Ast G, Woimant F, Georges B, Laurian C, Haguenau M: Spontaneous dissection of the internal carotid artery in 68 patients. Eur J Med 1993;2:466–472.
35 Steinke W, Rautenberg W, Schwartz A, Hennerici M: Noninvasive monitoring of internal carotid artery dissection. Stroke 1994;25:998–1005.
36 Brandt T, Stögbauer F, Ringelstein EB, Sitzer M: Dissektion hirnversorgender Arterien; in Diener HC, Hacke W, Forsting M (eds): Schlaganfall: Referenzreihe Neurologie – Klinische Neurologie. Stuttgart, New York, Thieme, 2004; pp 176–181.
37 Dreier JP, Lurtzing F, Kappmeier M, Bohner G, Klingebiel R, Leistner S, Einhaugl KM, Schielke E, Valdueza JM: Delayed occlusion after internal carotid artery dissection under heparin. Cerebrovasc Dis 2004;18:296–303.
38 Gubitz G, Sandercock P, Counsell C: Anticoagulants for acute ischaemic stroke. Cochrane Database Syst Rev 2004;(3):CD000024.
39 Biousse V, D'Anglejan-Chatillon J, Touboul PJ, Amarenco P, Bousser MG: Time course of symptoms in extracranial carotid artery dissections. A series of 80 patients. Stroke 1995;26:235–239.
40 Dziewas R, Konrad C, Drager B, Evers S, Besselmann M, Ludemann P, Kuhlenbaumer G, Stogbauer F, Ringelstein EB: Cervical artery dissection – Clinical features, risk factors, therapy and outcome in 126 patients. J Neurol 2003;250:1179–1184.
41 Youl BD, Coutellier A, Dubois B, Leger JM, Bousser MG: Three cases of spontaneous extracranial vertebral artery dissection. Stroke 1990;21:618–625.
42 Kaplan SS, Ogilvy CS, Gonzalez R, Gress D, Pile-Spellman J: Extracranial vertebral artery pseudoaneurysm presenting as subarachnoid hemorrhage. Stroke 1993;24:1397–1399.
43 Engelter ST, Lyrer PA, Kirsch EC, Steck AJ: Long-term follow-up after extracranial internal carotid artery dissection. Eur Neurol 2000;44:199–204.
44 Colella JJ, Diamond DL: Blunt carotid injury: Reassessing the role of anticoagulation. Am Surg 1996;62:212–217.
45 Marx A, Messing B, Storch B, Busse O: [Spontaneous dissection of arteries supplying the brain]. Nervenarzt 1987;58:8–18.
46 Chalmers TC, Celano P, Sacks HS, Smith H Jr: Bias in treatment assignment in controlled clinical trials. N Engl J Med 1983;309:1358–1361.
47 Wade DT: Measurements in Neurological Rehabilitation. Oxford, New York, Tokyo, Oxford University Press, 1992.
48 Biller J, Hingtgen WL, Adams HP Jr, Smoker WR, Godersky JC, Toffol GJ: Cervicocephalic arterial dissections. A ten-year experience. Arch Neurol 1986;43:1234–1238.
49 Biousse V, Schaison M, Touboul PJ, D'Anglejan-Chatillon J, Bousser MG: Ischemic optic neuropathy associated with internal carotid artery dissection. Arch Neurol 1998;55:715–719.
50 Bogousslavsky J, Despland PA, Regli F: Spontaneous carotid dissection with acute stroke. Arch Neurol 1987;44:137–140.
51 Chen ST, Ryu SJ, Hsi MS: Cervico-cerebral artery dissection. Taiwan Yi Xue Hui Za Zhi 1984;83:846–861.
52 de Bray JM, Dubas F, Joseph PA, Causeret H, Pasquier JP, Emile J: [Ultrasonic study of 22 cases of carotid artery dissection]. Rev Neurol (Paris) 1989;145:702–709.
53 Eachempati SR, Vaslef SN, Sebastian MW, Reed RL: Blunt vascular injuries of the head and neck: Is heparinization necessary? J Trauma 1998;45:997–1004.
54 Eljamel MS, Humphrey PR, Shaw MD: Dissection of the cervical internal carotid artery. The role of Doppler/Duplex studies and conservative management. J Neurol Neurosurg Psychiatry 1990;53:379–383.
55 Friedman WA, Day AL, Quisling RG, Sypert GW, Rhoton AL Jr: Cervical carotid dissecting aneurysms. Neurosurgery 1980;7:207–214.
56 Kaps M, Dorndorf W, Damian MS, Agnoli L: Intracranial haemodynamics in patients with spontaneous carotid dissection. Transcranial Doppler ultrasound follow-up studies. Eur Arch Psychiatry Neurol Sci 1990;239:246–256.

57 Landre E, Roux FX, Cioloca C: [Spontaneous dissection of the exocranial internal carotid artery. Therapeutic aspects]. Presse Med 1987;16:1273–1276.
58 Lepojarvi M, Tarkka M, Leinonen A, Kallanranta T: Spontaneous dissection of the internal carotid artery. Acta Chir Scand 1988;154;559–566.
59 Li MS, Smith BM, Espinosa J, Brown RA, Richardson P, Ford R: Nonpenetrating trauma to the carotid artery: Seven cases and a literature review. J Trauma 1994;36:265–272.
60 Luken MG III, Ascherl GF Jr, Correll JW, Hilal SK: Spontaneous dissecting aneurysms of the extracranial internal carotid artery. Clin Neurosurg 1979;26:353–375.
61 Fisher CM, Ojemann RG, Roberson GH: Spontaneous dissection of cervico-cerebral arteries. Can J Neurol Sci 1978;5:9–19.
62 Muller-Forell W, Rothacher G, Kramer G: [Carotid dissections]. Radiologe 1989;29:432–436.
63 Schievink WI, Limburg M: [Dissection of cervical arteries as a cause of cerebral ischemia or cranial nerve dysfunction]. Ned Tijdschr Geneeskd 1990;134:1843–1848.
64 Sellier N, Chiras J, Benhamou M, Bories J: Spontaneous dissection of the internal carotid artery. Clinical, radiologic and evolutive aspects. Apropos of 46 cases. J Neuroradiol 1983;10:243–259.
65 Vanneste JA, Davies G: Spontaneous dissection of the cervical internal carotid artery. Clin Neurol Neurosurg 1984;86:307–314.
66 Zelenock GB, Kazmers A, Whitehouse WM Jr, Graham LM, Erlandson EE, Cronenwett JL, Lindenauer SM, Stanely JC: Extracranial internal carotid artery dissections: Noniatrogenic traumatic lesions. Arch Surg 1982;117:425–432.
67 Schievink WI, Limburg M: [Dissection of cervical arteries as a cause of cerebral ischemia or cranial nerve dysfunction]. Ned Tijdschr Geneeskd 1990;134:1843–1848.
68 The Publications Committee for the Trial of ORG 10172 in Acute Stroke Treatment (TOAST) Investigators: Low molecular weight heparinoid, ORG 10172 (danaparoid), and outcome after acute ischemic stroke: A randomized controlled trial. JAMA 1998;279:1265–1272.
69 Adams HP Jr, Adams RJ, Brott T, del Zoppo GJ, Furlan A, Goldstein LB, Grubb RL, Higashida R, Kidwell C, Kwiatkowski TG, Marler JR, Hademenos GJ; Stroke Council of the American Stroke Association: Guidelines for the early management of patients with ischemic stroke: A scientific statement from the Stroke Council of the American Stroke Association. Stroke 2003;34:1056–1083.

Dr. Stefan Engelter
Neurological Clinic and Stroke Unit, University Hospital Basel
Petersgraben 4, CH–4031 Basel (Switzerland)
Tel. +41 61 265 25 25, Fax +41 61 265 56 44, E-Mail sengelter@uhbs.ch

Baumgartner RW, Bogousslavsky J, Caso V, Paciaroni M (eds): Handbook on Cerebral Artery Dissection. Front Neurol Neurosci. Basel, Karger, 2005, vol 20, pp 160–173

Intracranial Dissections

Michael Chen, Louis Caplan

Beth Israel Deaconess Medical Center, Department of Neurology, Division of Cerebrovascular Disease, Boston, Mass., USA

Abstract

Intracranial dissections have only been reported in small case series. More is known about the pathology, clinical findings, treatment and prognosis related to extracranial dissections. Knowing where within the arterial wall the dissection occurs is important in determining the appropriate treatment and prognosis. If the internal aspect of the artery is dissected, between the intima and media, vascular occlusion with resulting ischemia results. When the dissection plane is between the media and adventitia, bulging of the artery, with resultant aneurysmal dilatation, and vascular rupture can occur. In this chapter on intracranial dissections we will first review the pathology and etiology underlying intracranial dissections, then discuss the clinical aspects of both ischemic and aneurysmal intracranial dissections.

Intracranial arterial dissections have often been reported but the causes, clinical findings, angiographic features, and pathology are less well defined than in extracranial arterial dissections. When dissections involve the internal aspect of the arteries and extend between the intima and media, vascular occlusion with resulting ischemia is the predominant clinical picture. When the dissection plane is between the media and adventitia, bulging of the artery, with resultant aneurysmal dilatation, and vascular rupture often occur [1]. Despite sharing a similar mechanism for vascular disruption, the stark differences in presentation, treatment and prognosis must be distinguished. The literature on intracranial dissections is limited. With increased use of noninvasive cerebral vascular imaging, this finding may be detected with increasing frequency. In this review, we hope to better define this uncommon cause of stroke, such that the reader can be better informed to handle the challenging management questions that often accompany the patient with intracranial dissection.

Pathology

An intimal tear initiates dissection, allowing blood under arterial pressure to enter the wall of the artery. With extracranial arterial dissections being mostly medial, the thicker outer coats and supporting tissues probably prevent vascular rupture or limit extravascular bleeding [2]. In intracranial arteries, the absence of an external elastic lamina and a thin media and adventitia allows for subadventitial dissection and subsequent subarachnoid hemorrhage. The muscularis and adventitial layers of intracranial arteries are only about two thirds as thick as extracranial arteries, and lack well-developed external elastic membranes [3]. Vasa vasorum are diminished, which may limit healing intracranially [4]. The arterial dilation due to subadventitial dissections are often referred to as 'false aneurysms' or 'pseudoaneurysms', but should more accurately be referred to as 'dissecting aneurysms' because they do still contain all blood vessel elements. The thinner outer layers and weak supporting tissues of intracranial arteries probably explain their tendency to rupture. In 79% of the cases of intracranial dissection studied at necropsy by Yamaura and Ono [5], the plane of dissection in patients with subarachnoid hemorrhage lay between the media and the adventitia or within the media. The plane between the intima and media may be involved, leading to luminal compromise, often with thrombus formation and subsequent brain ischemia.

Among cases of intracranial dissection, the anterior circulation is more commonly involved in children and adolescents, whereas the posterior circulation is more often involved in adults [6]. Among adults, most posterior circulation intracranial dissections occur at the V4 segment at or near the origin of the posterior inferior cerebellar artery (PICA) [7]. The most commonly involved intracranial sites in the anterior circulation are the supraclinoid segment of the ICA and middle cerebral artery stem (fig. 1) [8]. An increasing number of dissections have been recognized to occur in the anterior cerebral artery (ACA). ACA dissections that manifest as ischemia typically involve the A2 portion, often with a double lumen or intimal flap. Those that present with hemorrhage tended to involve A1 dilatation with slight stenosis [9].

An intracranial dissection, once formed, is a dynamic pathological entity that fortunately usually changes to a more benign structure. Yamaura and Ono [5] operated on a dissecting aneurysm 36 days after onset and showed aneurysm organization. Intramural hematoma was seen in cases at 7, 17, and 28 days after onset. The other half of the cases showed dissections consisting of whitish gray, shiny and smooth surfaces regarded as complete organization of the hematoma. Dissections usually heal with time.

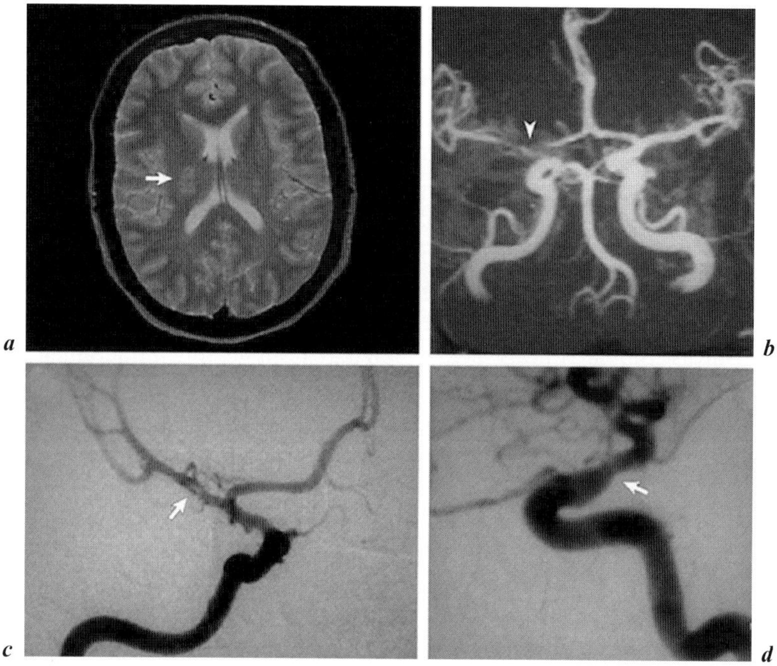

Fig. 1. ***a*** T2-weighted magnetic resonance imaging scan shows a right basal ganglia infarct. ***b*** Magnetic resonance angiography of the head demonstrates a filling defect (arrowhead) in the distal portion of the right ICA and proximal middle cerebral artery stem. Cerebral angiography shows the presence of double lumen in the right MCA stem (***c***, arrow) and narrowing of the supraclinoid portion of the right ICA (***d***, arrow) [8].

Mizutani et al. [10] showed that the pattern of intimal injury determined the risk for rehemorrhage. Lesions were categorized as either entrance only (fig. 2) or having a communication through the intima with the aneurysm (fig. 3). Entrance-only lesions appeared to have a higher occurrence of bleeding implicating the effects of constant pressure and pulsation on the lesion.

Epidemiology

Intracranial dissection is an under-diagnosed cause for stroke among younger patients. A review of 59 intracranial carotid dissection cases showed the mean age at onset to be 30 years of age with a male preponderance [11]. In another series of vertebral dissection associated with subarachnoid hemorrhage, the average age was 49.6 years and two thirds were men [12]. Koyama et al. [13] suggest that the observed male predominance may reflect intimal

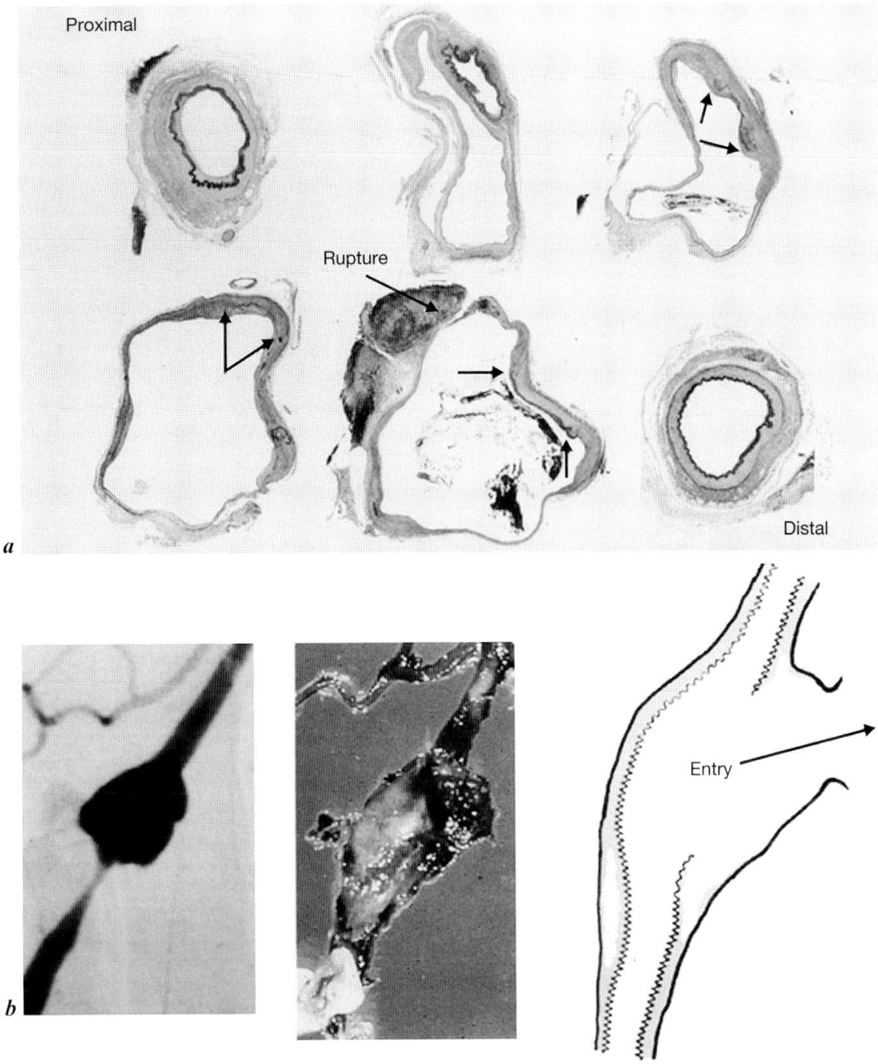

Fig. 2. ***a*** Photomicrograph showing serial axial slices of a typical entry-only dissecting aneurysm treated conservatively and removed 35 days post-subarachnoid hemorrhage. The wall adjacent to the rupture site (long arrow) is only composed of fibrin and thin collagen. Elastica van Gieson, original magnification ×40. ***b*** Right vertebral artery angiogram (left) revealing a fusiform aneurysm with an irregular contour. Photograph (center) of the aneurysm, obtained at autopsy on day 35 post-subarachnoid hemorrhage. Illustration (right) of the reconstructed entry-only dissecting aneurysm. Wavy line represents the internal elastic lamina; gray area represents the media [10].

a

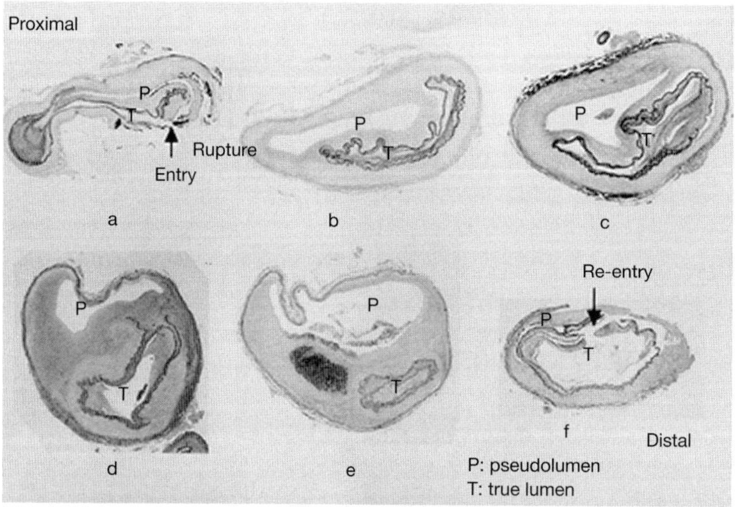

b

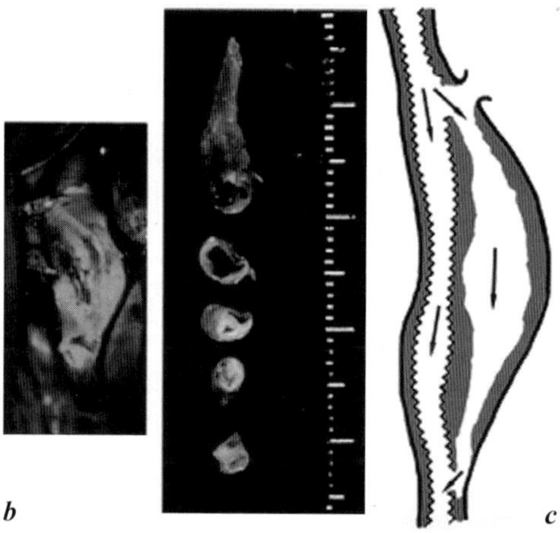

c

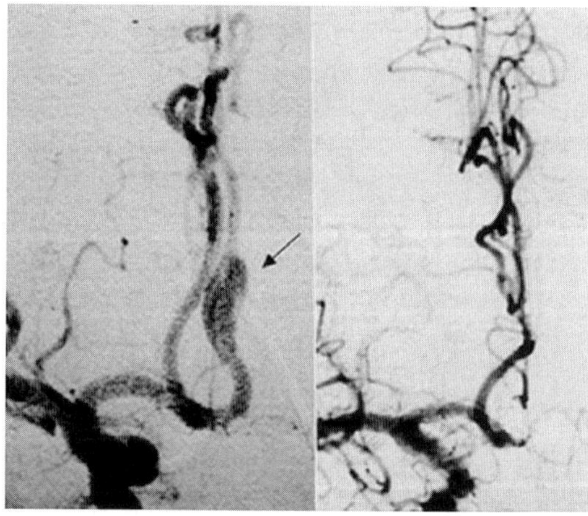

Fig. 3. ***a*** Photomicrograph demonstrating serial axial slices (a–f) of an entry-exit dissecting aneurysm. Elastica van Gieson, original magnification ×40. ***b*** Intraoperative photograph of the aneurysm (left), serial sections of the aneurysm (center), and illustration of a reconstructed entry-exit dissecting aneurysm (right). Wavy line represents the internal elastic lamina and gray area represents the media. ***c*** Preoperative right carotid artery angiogram (left) with fusiform aneurysm with smooth contour (arrow) and postoperative right carotid angiogram (right) confirming successful A3–A3 bypass [10].

fibroelastic abnormalities related to sex hormones. Dissecting aneurysms of the vertebrobasilar system accounts for 3–7% of subarachnoid hemorrhage cases [14]. On the contrary, subarachnoid hemorrhage is reported in about one fifth of intracranial ICA dissections and in more than half of intracranial vertebral artery dissections [6]. The higher incidence in younger patients is an important epidemiological feature that can aid in the diagnosis of this uncommon, non-specific pathology.

Etiology

The cause of intracranial arterial dissection remains unknown. Activities associated with mechanical stretching of the arteries is associated with extracranial arterial dissection but has not been well studied in intracranial dissections. Theoretically, there is less mobility and contact with bony structures as compared with the extracranial cervical arteries. The dura anchors the vertebral artery as it enters intracranially. One of the authors has, however, personally seen cases of intracranial dissection in a volleyball player and a fireman, where there was a clear history of preceding head trauma.

An underlying arteriopathy may lead to structural instability of the vessel wall increasing the susceptibility to intimal tear. Of the heritable connective tissue disorders most strongly associated with spontaneous dissection is Ehlers-Danlos syndrome type IV [15]. Fibromuscular dysplasia is found in 15–20% of all patients with cervicocephalic dissection and in half of those with bilateral carotid involvement [16]. Other associated disorders only found in a small percentage of dissection cases include Marfan's syndrome, autosomal dominant polycystic kidney disease, and osteogenesis imperfecta type I [15]. Migraine is more common in patients with dissection and is thought to be mediated by edema of the vessel wall during a migraine attack that makes it vulnerable to tear. Those patients with pre-existing defects in the vessel wall are more likely to have multiple extensive dissections and have associated subarachnoid hemorrhage.

Autopsy studies have not identified pre-existing defects on routine examination of the arteries. Fibromuscular dysplasia and cystic medial necrosis are common findings on postmortem examination but are nonspecific and associated with a variety of systemic disorders. Some patients have perivascular inflammation. However, similar changes are seen in patients with subarachnoid hemorrhage without dissection and may be due to the hemorrhage. Ultrastructural abnormalities of dermal connective tissue components have been detected in two thirds of patients with spontaneous dissection in cervicocephalic arteries. No mutation in the gene for type III procollagen (COL2A1), type V procollagen (COL5A1) or tropoelastin (ELN) has been identified [10].

Clinical and Diagnostic Features

Acute Ischemia

One of the first descriptions of intracranial dissections came from Scholefield [17], who, in 1924 reported a case of a 47-year-old man who had headache, neck pain, and nausea followed 3 days later by right facial weakness and left hemiplegia. At necropsy a dissection of the right intracranial vertebral artery extending into the basilar artery was found.

Severe unilateral headache is almost universally present, and ischemic symptoms typically occur with a much shorter delay as compared with extracranial dissections [18]. In extracranial ICA dissection for example, initial symptoms may precede the stroke by several days [19]. Another distinction of extracranial ICA dissection is that it may be associated with vigorous activity, a Horner's syndrome, or pulsatile tinnitus without cerebral ischemia, whereas patients with intracranial dissection usually have brain ischemia and no history of vigorous activity [12, 20]. Fluctuation of neurological signs during the first 2 weeks after symptom onset is also more characteristic of dissections occurring intracranially. In contrast to distal embolism, the mechanism thought to be responsible in extracranial dissection, cerebral hypoperfusion, is likely a primary mechanism explaining fluctuating neurological signs [19].

In the anterior circulation, three quarters of instances involve the more distal, supraclinoid segment of the ICA stem; the ACA is less often involved [6, 7] (fig. 4). Giant cell arteritis may be confused with distal ICA dissection [20]. However, giant cell arteritis usually involves the petrous and cavernous segments of the ICA, affects a much older population and is associated with an increased erythrocyte sedimentation rate [21].

In the posterior circulation, the intracranial vertebral artery is most often involved at or near the PICA junction, often extending into the basilar artery. Primary basilar artery dissections are less common. Intracranial vertebral artery dissection can cause brainstem infarction with an associated high morbidity and mortality. Often, the initial signs suggest a unilateral brainstem lesion [22]. Headache remains a prominent symptom even in posterior circulation dissection [12].

An aggressive diagnostic approach is immediately warranted when ischemia due to arterial dissection is clinically suggested. Conventional angiography remains the mainstay in accurately defining the exact location and arterial territory of the intracranial dissection. String sign, double lumen, irregular scalloped stenosis, and vessel occlusion are usually seen when the dissection involves the subintimal and intramedial layers [20].

MRI may be practically useful in the noninvasive diagnosis of both extra- and intracranial dissection. In the subacute stage, dissection appears as a

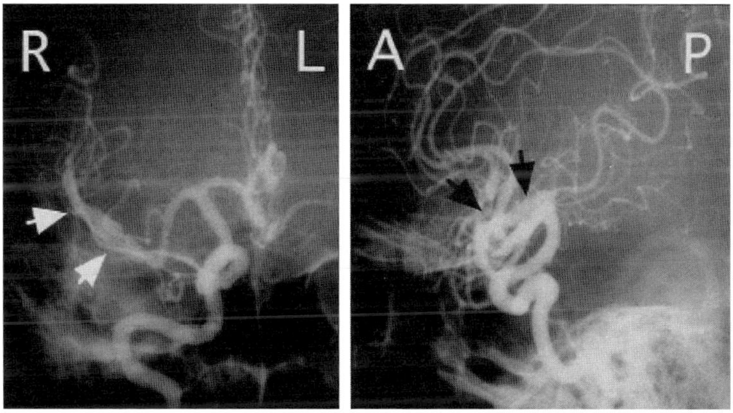

Fig. 4. AP (left) and lateral (right) views: Right carotid angiogram demonstrating an irregularity and bulbous dilatation of the right M2 [24].

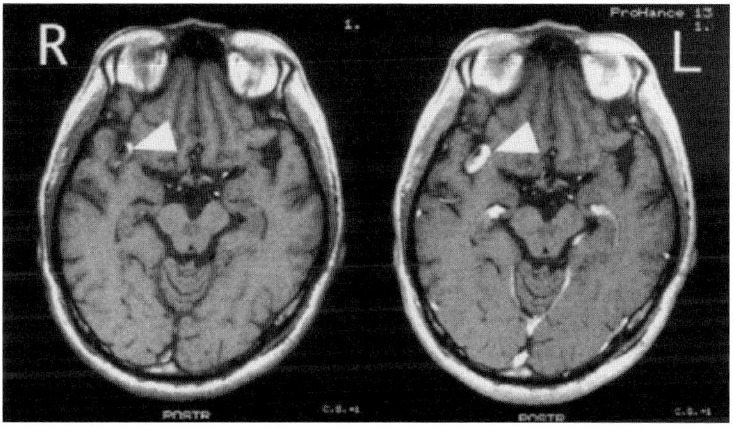

Fig. 5. Axial MR image revealing a high-intensity area and crescent enhancement with contrast medium around a dilated signal void of the right M2 (arrow) (left: T1-weighted image, right: T1-weighted image with contrast medium) [24].

hyperintense crescentic intramural signal on T1- and T2-weighted cross-section images correlating with an intramural hematoma (fig. 5) [18].

Chronic Ischemia

Chronic, large dissecting aneurysms can harbor thrombi, which later serve as a source for intra-arterial embolism. Caplan et al. [12] described a case of a 33-year-old woman with multiple posterior circulation transient ischemic attacks and small strokes. Bilateral carotid and left vertebral angiograms showed a large dissecting aneurysm of the left intracranial vertebral artery with luminal filling defect thought to represent an intimal flap or a thrombus. She demonstrated a dramatic response to the combination of aspirin and a warfarin analog, suggesting the mechanism of her repeated ischemia was intra-arterial embolism of platelet-fibrin-thrombin aggregates.

Large or strategically located dissecting aneurysms can also compress local brain structures and cranial nerves [1]. De Busscher [23] described a 45-year-old man with a 4-month history of progressive disability beginning with severe head and neck ache followed by vertigo, dysphagia, staggering, and unilateral face and limb paresthesias. Necropsy revealed a large left vertebral artery dissecting aneurysm compressing the lower brainstem and cranial nerves. Kurino et al. [24] described a case of a 45-year-old man with mild left flaccid paresis that worsened after 8 days, diagnosed by MRI to be a right M2 dissecting aneurysm. About 2 months afterwards, he developed transient worsening of left-sided weakness and was found to have progressive changes in the right M2 dilatation. Fortunately though, conservative treatment with antihypertensive and antiplatelet medications were continued and follow-up angiography 6 months afterwards demonstrated no further progression of the right M2 dilatation. He had then been followed with serial MRI/angiograms without changes and a satisfactory clinical course.

Subarachnoid Hemorrhage

Headache due to subarachnoid hemorrhage is the major clinical presentation of patients with dissecting intracranial aneurysms. Neck pain may be prominent but location, severity, and radiation of the pain is, as expected, nonspecific and not different from aneurysmal bleeding in patients without dissection.

In 1977, Yonas et al. [3] first described the major diagnostic angiographic findings of dissecting aneurysms to be an irregular vessel lumen with proximal narrowing. Other markers include a fusiform dilation and proximal and/or distal narrowing ('pearl-and-string' sign), double lumen, irregular scalloped stenosis, and retention of contrast medium in the venous phase [25, 26]. The double lumen is the only truly diagnostic sign of a dissecting aneurysm [5]. Distinguishing dissecting aneurysms from true aneurysms and simple dissections enable proper treatment. Finding an aneurysmal formation at a nonbifurcation location in the context of subarachnoid hemorrhage suggests dissection rather than aneurysm (fig. 4). In the posterior circulation, aneurysmal dilation of the intracranial vertebral artery most often occurs at or near the PICA junction. There is often narrowing of the artery proximal or distal to the aneurysm, often attributed before operation to 'vasospasm'. Dissecting aneurysms with a pearl-and-string structure presenting with subarachnoid hemorrhage are associated with a poor outcome, and may be candidates for aggressive intervention if they present with favorable Hunt and Kosnik grades [27].

In addition to the location and configuration of the dissecting aneurysm, other important features to determine on angiography include identifying adjacent branches, collateral circulation, and the time course [10].

MRI is quite useful in the noninvasive diagnosis of both extra- and intracranial dissecting aneurysms. In the subacute stage, dissection appears as a hyperintense crescentic intramural signal on T1- and T2-weighted images correlating with an intramural hematoma [28]. Nagahiro et al. [29] noted distinct enhancement of dissecting aneurysms on gadolinium-enhanced MRI in all patients whose angiograms showed aneurysm dilation or pearl-and-string signs. Presence of subarachnoid hemorrhage suggests intracranial extension of extracranial vertebral artery dissection. Intracranial vertebral artery dissection occurs near the origin of the PICA. Again, noninvasive imaging can only suggest the diagnosis when associated with subarachnoid hemorrhage. Angiography is usually warranted in these cases. However, once established, primarily because the management of vertebrobasilar dissecting aneurysms remains controversial, conservatively treated patients should be examined repeatedly with MRI to establish the dynamic course of the lesion [29].

Treatment

Cerebral ischemia caused by intracranial dissection without subarachnoid hemorrhage is usually mediated by focal cerebral hypoperfusion and less often by artery-to-artery embolism [18]. Because of the speculated propensity of intracranial dissections to bleed, anticoagulation is typically avoided. If the stroke mechanism is thought to be due to thromboembolism, Schievink [30] recommend antiplatelet therapy with serial MRI/angiograms every 3 months for a year, with antiplatelet discontinuation if there is normalization of the affected vessel [30]. The 3-month duration of therapy is arbitrary and imaging studies confirming recanalization is probably indicated before any change in therapy. Careful follow-up is mandatory before contemplating treatment modalities with potential serious side effects. As described above, the pathological evidence of whitish gray, shiny smooth surface of the hematoma coupled with the rather rapid angiographic improvement suggest that arterial dissection eventually cures itself.

There has been some controversy over the use of intravenous thrombolysis in acute stroke patients with dissection suggested on history or examination. There is the theoretical risk of causing increased hemorrhage into the vessel wall. Despite only 30 reported cases, tissue plasminogen activator given both intravenously and intra-arterially had been administered safely after cervicocephalic-arterial-dissection-related stroke [31]. Some advocate using intra-arterial rather than intravenous thrombolysis to avoid the above-mentioned risk. They recommend placing the catheter tip in the distal thrombus, beyond the site of dissection, thereby minimizing the exposure of torn intima to the thrombolytic agent [18].

Neuroendovascular intervention is considered in patients for whom medical therapy has failed and who have persistent ischemic symptoms, limited reserve due to involvement of other vessels, or persistent or expanding dissecting aneurysm. Neuroendovascular intervention is most often considered when the stroke mechanism is thought to be due to hemodynamic compromise. Extracranially, these techniques allow for re-establishment of the true lumen and obliteration of the false lumen, reducing the risk of artery-to-artery embolism. The majority of the interventions for dissection have been performed in the extracranial circulation. Sequential reconstruction of the true lumen is accomplished by means of stents that provide gradual radial force, permitting apposition of the dissected segment to the vessel wall. Because the risk of recurrent embolization is low, stenting as an initial therapy is not warranted and should be reserved in most cases for those that fail medical therapy [32].

Anticoagulation is clearly contraindicated in cases of dissecting aneurysms with subarachnoid hemorrhage. These patients should be medically managed similar to a patient with the more common aneurysmal subarachnoid hemorrhage.

Surgical ligation or coil embolization to occlude the affected segment of artery is often the preferred therapy for vertebral artery dissecting aneurysms. Irie et al. [26] published a series of case reports of intracranial dissecting aneurysms treated with angioplasty and coils held in place with stents. A trapping procedure is the most complete treatment for a dissecting aneurysm but comes with the risk of side branch occlusion, potentially further injuring the vessel wall or dislodging emboli [33].

Occasionally, complex surgical procedures such as saphenous/radial artery bypass or PICA side-to-side reanastomosis are employed [33]. But in general, surgical treatment for symptomatic dissecting aneurysm or postdissection stenosis has decreased. Aneurysmal clipping is usually not an option because of the typically fusiform configuration.

Medically refractory cases of intracranial vertebral artery dissection have been most recently treated with balloon occlusion if temporary occlusion studies suggest adequate collateral blood flow [18]. Proximal occlusion has the advantage of limiting the risk of catheter and wire manipulation across the narrow or irregular segment and may allow for better collateral circulation. Lesions involving the PICA origin or anterior spinal artery are most amenable. The configuration of certain dissecting aneurysms (fusiform or wide-neck) may not hold coils in a stable position and would hence be more appropriately occluded proximally [33].

Prognosis

The initial reported cases of intracranial vertebral artery dissections were invariably fatal [12]. This was not surprising given that most cases were diagnosed during autopsy. As would be expected though with more widespread use of noninvasive cerebrovascular imaging, intracranial dissections with milder clinical syndromes are being detected. More recent case series demonstrate a far more favorable outcome than previously thought. In a study by Yamada et al. [27] of 24 patients with vertebral artery dissection treated conservatively, those with lesions appearing stenotic or occlusive on angiogram had good outcomes. In series of Chaves et al. [20] of 10 patients with intracranial ICA dissection, 6 of who received immediate anticoagulation, all did well with no to moderate disability at 3 months. In the group of ACA dissections collected, all cases seen in follow-up showed serial improvement of the stenotic portion and improvement by 2 months. These results support the suspected dynamic nature of these lesions. In practical terms, if the initial diagnostic angiogram shows an aneurysm of unclear etiology, seeing serial improvement on follow-up studies, spaced months apart, can suggest dissection rather than true aneurysm [9]. Kitanaka et al. [34] followed 6 cases of intracranial vertebral artery dissection without subarachnoid hemorrhage and felt that if there was improving angiographic follow-up, nonsurgical, supportive care focused on bed rest, withholding antithrombotics and blood pressure control was most appropriate. Yamada et al. [27] followed 24 patients with vertebral artery dissection who were treated conservatively. Rebleeding and short insult-to-admission intervals were strongly associated with poor outcomes.

References

1 Caplan LR: Posterior Circulation Disease. Cambridge, Blackwell Publishers, 1996, pp 284–291.
2 O'Connell BF, Towfighi J, Brennan RW: Dissecting aneurysms of the head and neck. Neurology 1985;35:993–997.
3 Yonas H, Agamonolis D, Takaoka Y, White RJ: Dissecting intracranial aneurysms. Surg Neurol 1977;8:407–415.
4 Scott G, Neuberger K, Denst J: Dissecting aneurysms of the intracranial arteries. Neurology 1960; 10:22–27.
5 Yamaura A, Ono J: Current diagnosis and treatment of intracranial dissecting aneurysms. Neurosurg Q 1994;4:67–81.

6 Schievink WI, Mokri B, Jackers G: Spontaneous dissections of cervicocephalic arteries in childhood and adolesence. Neurology 1994;44:1607–1612.
7 Mokri B, Houser OW, Sandock BA, Piepgras DG: Spontaneous dissection of the vertebral arteries. Neurology 1988;38:880–885.
8 Chaves C, Estol C, Esnaola M, Gorson K, O'Donoghue, DeWitt LD, Caplan LR: Spontaneous intracranial internal carotid artery dissection. Arch Neurol 2002;59:977–981.
9 Ohkuma H, Suzuki S, Kikkawa T, Shimamura N: Neuroradiologic and clinical features of arterial dissection of the anterior cerebral artery. AJNR A J Neuroradiol 2003;24:691–699.
10 Mizutani T, Kojima H, Asamoto S, Miki Y: Pathologic mechanism and three-dimensional structure of cerebral dissecting aneurysms. J Neurosurg 2001;94:712–717.
11 Bassetti C, Bogousslavsky J, Eskenasy-Cottier AC: Spontaneous intracranial dissection in the anterior circulation. Cerebrovasc Dis 1994;4:170.
12 Caplan LR, Baquis GD, Pessin MS, D'Alton J, Adelman LS, DeWitt LD, Ho K, Izukawa D, Kwan ES: Dissection of the intracranial vertebral artery. Neurology 1988;38:868–877.
13 Koyama S, Kotani A, Sasaki J: Spontaneous dissecting aneurysm of the anterior cerebral artery: Report of two cases. Surg Neurol 1996;46:55–61.
14 Rabinov J, Hellinger F, Morris P, Ogilvy C, Putman C: Endovascular management of vertebrobasilar dissecting aneurysms. AJNR A J Neuroradiol 2003;24:1421–1428.
15 Schievink WI, Michels VV, Piepgras DG: Neurovascular manifestations of heritable connective tissue disorders: A review. Stroke 1994;25:889–903.
16 Schievink WI, Mokri B, O'Fallon M: Recurrent spontaneous cervical artery dissection. N Engl J Med 1994;330:393–397.
17 Scholefield BG: A case of aneurysm of the basilar artery. Guys Hosp Rep 1924;4:485–487.
18 Mohr JP, Choi DW, Grotta JC, Weir B, Wolf PA: Stroke: Pathophysiology, Diagnosis, and Management, ed 4. Philadelphia, Pa., Churchill Livingstone, 2004, pp 549–573.
19 Hart RG, Easton JD: Dissections of cervical and cerebral arteries. Neurol Clin 1983;1:155–182.
20 Chaves C, Estol C, Esnaola M, Gorson K, O'Donoghue, DeWitt LD, Caplan LR: Spontaneous intracranial internal carotid artery dissection. Arch Neurol 2002;59:977–981.
21 Wildinson IM, Russel RW: Arteries of the head and neck in giant cell arteritis: A pathological study to show the pattern of arterial involvement. Arch Neurol 1972;27:378–391.
22 Fukuda M, Aiba T, Takahashi S: Bilateral medial medullary infarction due to bilateral vertebral artery dissection. Clin Neurol Neurosurg 2004;106:132–135.
23 De Busscher J: Aneurysme de l'artere vertebrale gauche chez un homme 45 ans. Acta Neurol Psychiatr Belg 1952;52:1–23.
24 Kurino M, Yoshioka S, Yukitaka U: Spontaneous dissecting aneurysms of the anterior and middle cerebral artery associated with brain infarction. Surg Neurol 2002;57:428–437.
25 Kunze S, Schiefer W: Angiographic demonstration of a dissecting aneurysm of the middle cerebral artery. Neuroradiology 1971;2:201–206.
26 Irie K, Negoro M, Hayakawa M, Hayashi J, Kanno T: Treatment of spontaneous intracranial dissecting aneurysm with stent-assisted coil embolization. Neuroradiology 2003;45:835–829.
27 Yamada M, Kitahara T, Kurata A, Fujii K, Miyasaka Y: Intracranial vertebral artery dissection with subarachnoid hemorrhage: Clinical characteristics and outcomes in conservatively treated patients. J Neurosurg 2004;101:25–30.
28 Brugieres P, Castrec-Carpo A, Heran F, Goujon C, Gaston A, Marsault C: Magnetic resonance imaging in the exploration of dissection of the internal carotid artery. J Neuroradiol 1989;16:1–10.
29 Nagahiro S, Hamada J, Sakamoto Y, Ushio Y: Follow-up evaluation of dissecting aneurysms of the vertebrobasilar circulation by using gadolinium-enhanced magnetic resonance imaging. J Neurosurg 1997;87:385–390.
30 Schievink WI: Spontaneous dissection of the carotid and vertebral arteries. N Engl J Med 2001; 344:898–906.
31 Derex L, Nighoghossian N, Turjman F, Hermier M, Honnorat J, Neuschwander P, Froment JC, Trouillas P: Intravenous tPA in acute ischemic stroke related to internal carotid artery dissection. Neurology 2000;54:2159–2161.
32 Schievink WI: The treatment of spontaneous carotid and vertebral artery dissections. Curr Opin Cardiol 2000;15:318.

33 Takikawa S, Kamiyama H, Nomura M, Abe H, Saitoh H: Vertebral dissecting aneurysms treated with trapping and bilateral PICA side-to-side anastomosis: A case report. Neurol Surg 1991;19: 571–576.
34 Kitanaka C, Tanaki J, Kuwahara M, Teraoka A, Sasaki T, Takakura K: Nonsurgical treatment of unruptured intracranial vertebral artery dissection with serial follow-up angiography. J Neurosurg 1994;80:667–674.

Michael Chen, MD
Beth Israel Deaconess Medical Center
Department of Neurology
Division of Cerebrovascular Disease
330 Brookline Avenue
Palmer 132
Boston, MA 02215 (USA)
Tel. +1 617 632 8911, Fax +1 617 632 8920, E-Mail chenm888@yahoo.com

Author Index

Subject Index